Plant-Based Manual

Lose weight and stay fit with the Plant-Based recipe Manual!

Carolyn J. Perez

This Book Included

Book 1:

PLANT-BASED DIET FOR BEGINNERS

Easy and tasty recipes for every day to lose weight.

Book 2:

A PLANT-BASED DIET COOKBOOK

Lose weight and stay fit with easy and delicious Plant-Based recipes.

Carolyn J. Perez

Plant-Based Diet for beginners

Easy and tasty recipes for every day to lose weight

Carolyn J. Perez

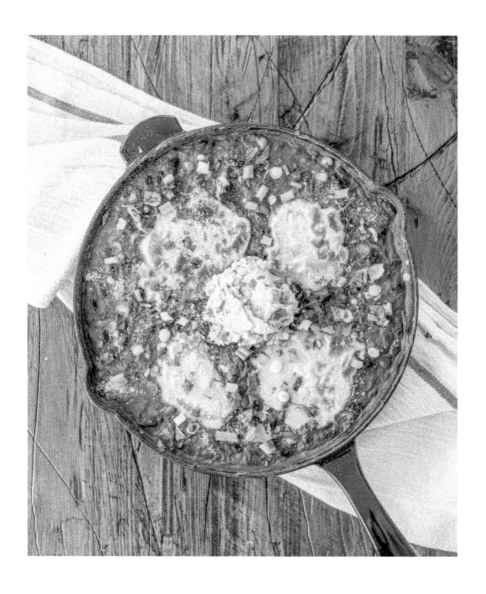

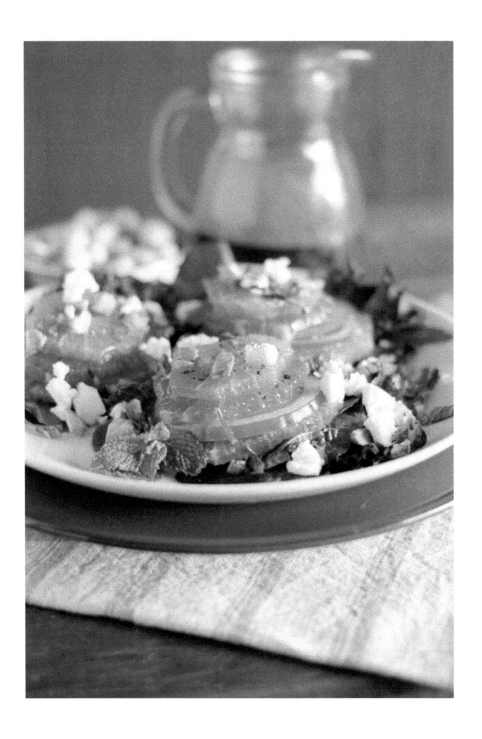

Contents

INTRODUCTION.. 10

PLANT BASED DIET: WHAT ARE WE TALKING ABOUT?.................. 12

MAIN DIFFERENCES BETWEEN VEGAN AND PLANT BASED DIET
.... 13

SIDE DISHES RECIPES.. 22
    Lime pine nuts and fennel salad 22
    Orange chickpeas and fennel salad 24
    Cucumber soy yogurt salad 25
    Lettuce and cauliflower salad with tofu... 26
    Belgian endive salad with orange.. 28
    Brussels salad.. 29
    Alsatian salad.. 31
    Onions and bell peppers salad... 33
    Mushrooms and green olives salad 34
    Country salad 36
    Green beans potatoes and tofu salad 37
    Avocado salad... 38
    Red cabbage and hazelnuts salad.. 41
    Green beans onions and almond cheese.. 43
    Vegetable salad with mayonnaise 44
    Summer salad with soy yogurt 45
    Escarole citrus salad 48
    Grand duke Salad 50
    Asparagus and hazelnuts salad 52
    Stuffed mushrooms turnips 53
    Cream of cucumbers.. 55
    Basil zucchini.. 57
    Zucchini with rice sauce.. 59
    Sweet & Sour vegetables... 61
    Zucchini with mushrooms and parsley... 64
    Marinated zucchini.. 66
    Baked zucchini with béchamel... 68
    Cabbage rolls 69
    Cabbage and potato soup 70
    Leeks soup... 72
    Leeks and onions croquettes... 74
    Aromatic potato salad... 76
    Pineapple and celery salad 78

Flavoured fennel and leeks *79*
Oven-roasted tomatoes *81*
Golden zucchini *82*
Onions with mustard sauce *83*
Gratin onions *84*
Pumpkin glazed with soy and sesame *85*
Pan-fried mushrooms and beans *86*
Ratatouille *88*
DESSERT AND FRUIT RECIPES *91*
Chocolate and vanilla bread *91*
Chocolate coconut and pistachios bread *93*
Soy and Apple bread with chocolate *95*
Coconut and apple bread *97*
Raspberry and soy bread *99*
Strawberry ginger bread *101*
Cinnamon and vanilla bread *103*
Coconut and vanilla bread *105*
Almond and soy bread *107*
Orange and almond bread *109*

Introduction

It is a common thought to think that following a diet is necessarily linked to the concept of actual weight loss. However, this is not always the case: following a diet is often directly linked to the foods that we decide to include in our tables daily.

In addition, we do not always choose the best quality ingredients to cook our dishes.

Sometimes we are so rushed and unruly that we forget that we love our bodies. And what better cure than a healthy diet? Following a healthy diet should become more than an imposition or a punishment, but a real lifestyle.

Moreover, this is the Plant-based diet goal: not to impose a restrictive and sometimes impossible diet to follow, but to recreate a diet based on foods of natural origin and above all healthy. Therefore, the plant based represents a real food trend. However, as we will see it is much more than just a fashion trend, but a real lifestyle.

In addition, it is the aim of this text, or rather of this cookbook, to introduce you to the plant based discipline. And we will do it with a few theoretical explanations, just to make you understand what we are talking about and above all how to prepare it: there will be a purely practical part where you will find 800 recipes on the plant based. These recipes will be divided into appetizers, snacks, first and second courses, side dishes and finally a string of plant based desserts.

In the end, you will be spoiled for choice to start following this healthy dietary discipline.

Plant based diet: what are we talking about?

We already mentioned that more than a real weight loss diet the Plant based diet is a food discipline. Food discipline is enjoying great success not only because it is very fashionable, but because it applies such principles that can be perfectly integrated into our daily lives. The plant-based diet is a true approach to life, starting with nutrition: respect for one's health and body, first of all, which is reflected in respect for all forms of life and the planet in general.

As the word itself says, it deals with a food plan based, precisely on what comes from plants. However, simply calling it that way would be too simplistic.

It is a predominantly plant-based diet, but not only. It is not just about consuming vegetables but about taking natural foods: not industrially processed, not treated, and not deriving from the exploitation of resources and animals, preferably zero km.

So it could be a discipline that aims not only at environmental saving but also at the economic one: think about what advantages, in fact, at the level of your pockets you can have if you apply the principle of 0Km and therefore to be able to harvest your vegetables directly from your garden.

Environmental savings do not only mean pollution reduction: the ethical component (present exclusively in the vegan diet, for example) is combined with a strong will to health. This means that the plant based, in addition to not preferring foods that exploit animals, is also based on foods that are especially unprocessed, fresh, healthy, balanced, light, and rich in essential nutrients. In practice, it is a plant-based diet but not vegan / vegetarian, emphasizing the quality and wholesomeness of foods rather than on their moral value, albeit with great attention to sustainability. Such a lifestyle could therefore be of help, not only to our health, but also to create a more sustainable world for future generations.

Main differences between Vegan and Plant based diet

The plant-based diet is often associated with the vegan diet. This is because both plan to include cruelty free foods that do not involve any animal exploitation.

Furthermore, they are associated precisely because they are both predominantly plant-based.

However, there are some pretty obvious differences between these two diets.

First of all, precisely for the reasoning behind the prevalence of plants.

It is well known that even the vegan diet provides a diet based on foods of plant origin: unlike the plant-based diet, however, nothing of animal derivation is allowed, neither direct nor indirect, nor other products - clothing or accessories - which include the exploitation of animals.

No eggs, no milk, no honey, no leather, so to speak, and not only: in its most rigorous meanings, veganism does not even include the use of yeasts, as the bacteria that compose them are indisputably living beings.

A vegan diet can be balanced if the person who leads it knows well the foods and their combinations, the necessary supplements, and their body's reaction to the lack of certain foods.

On the contrary, the Plant-Based diet is on the one hand more relaxed, on the other more stringent.

What does it mean?

This means that it is on the one hand more relaxed because it is plant-based, but not exclusively vegetable: products of animal origin are allowed, in moderate quantities, but under only one condition, namely the excellent quality of the food itself and its certified origin. For example, eggs can be consumed occasionally but only if very fresh, possibly at zero km, from free-range farms where the hens are not exploited but can live outdoors without constraints.

It is also a somewhat more stringent philosophy than veganism precisely for this reason: as long as it is 100% vegetable, the vegan also consumes heavily processed foods, such as industrial fries. Therefore, the vegan can also eat junk foods or snacks. Conversely, plant-based dieters would never admit highly refined foods of this type.

Both dietary approaches are conscious and do not involve the consumption of meat. However, if vegans are driven by ethical reasons, those who follow a plant-based diet also reject everything processed on an industrial level and unhealthy.

A plant-based diet is a diet that aims to eliminate industrially processed foods and, therefore, potentially more harmful to health. It is based on the consumption of fruit and vegetables, whole grains and avoiding (or minimizing) animal products and processed foods. This means that vegan desserts made with refined sugar or bleached flour are also covered.

There is also a substantial difference between the philosophies behind the two diets. As we said in the previous paragraph and above, the ethical component, which is based on the refusal of any food of animal origin, plays a lot in veganism. While for the plant based is not a purely moral and moralistic discourse but on the real thought of being able to keep healthy with the food discipline and be respectful of the environment surrounding us.

Plant based diet full shopping list. What to eat and what to avoid

Now we can examine the complete shopping list of the plant based diet.

Let's briefly summarize the principles on which this particular type of diet is based:

- Emphasizes whole, minimally processed foods.
- Limits or avoids animal products.
- Focuses on plants, including vegetables, fruits, whole grains, legumes, seeds and nuts, which should make up most of what you eat.
- Excludes refined foods, like added sugars, white flour and processed oils.
- Pays special attention to food quality, promoting locally sourced, organic food whenever possible.

As for what you can usually eat, we can say the general consumption of:

- Wholegrain and flours
- extra virgin olive oil

- Seasonal fruit and vegetables: these foods are the basis of every meal.
- In this diet you can also eat sweets but only and exclusively homemade and with controlled raw materials, simple and not very refined, preferably of vegetable origin - for example by replacing milk with soy or rice drinks, and eggs with other natural thickeners such as flaxseed, or simple ripe banana.
- You can also consume nuts and seeds.

As for absolutely forbidden foods, there are all those ready-made and processed:

- ready-made sauces
- chips
- biscuits
- various kinds of snacks
- sugary cereals,
- Spreads, snacks and many other notoriously unhealthy foods.
- Junk food and fast food are therefore absolutely banned
- Sugar beverages

Regarding the complete shopping list:

- Fruits: Berries, citrus fruits, pears, peaches, pineapple, bananas, etc.

- Vegetables: Kale, spinach, tomatoes, broccoli, cauliflower, carrots, asparagus, peppers, etc.

- Starchy vegetables: Potatoes, sweet potatoes, butternut squash, etc.

- Whole grains: Brown rice, rolled oats, spelt, quinoa, brown rice pasta, barley, etc.

- Healthy fats with omega 3: Avocados, olive oil, coconut oil, unsweetened coconut, etc.

- Legumes: Peas, chickpeas, lentils, peanuts, beans, black beans, etc.

- Seeds, nuts and nut butter: Almonds, cashews, macadamia nuts, pumpkin seeds, sunflower seeds, natural peanut butter, tahini, etc.

- Unsweetened plant-based milk: Coconut milk, almond milk, cashew milk, etc.

- Spices, herbs and seasonings: Basil, rosemary, turmeric, curry, black pepper, salt, etc.

- Condiments: Salsa, mustard, nutritional yeast, soy sauce, vinegar, lemon juice, etc.

- Plant-based protein: Tofu, tempeh, seitan, and plant based protein sources or powders with no added sugar or artificial ingredients.
- Beverages: Coffee, tea, sparkling water, etc.

There is the chance to add food of animal origin very rarely, for example if you have specific nutritional needs or if it has been strongly recommended by your doctor. Anyway, if supplementing your plant-based diet with animal products choose quality products from grocery stores or, better yet, purchase them from local farms.

- Eggs: Pasture-raised when possible.
- Poultry: Free-range, organic when possible.
- Beef and pork: Pastured or grass-fed when possible.
- Seafood: Wild-caught from sustainable fisheries when possible.
- Dairy: Organic dairy products from pasture-raised animals whenever possible.

Side dishes recipes

Lime pine nuts and fennel salad

PREPARATION TIME: 10 minutes
COOKING TIME: 30 minutes
CALORIES: 125

INGREDIENTS FOR 4 SERVINGS

- 2 fennels
- 2 lime
- The juice of half a lime
- a spoonful of curry
- 6 tablespoons of oil
- 2 shallots (or two small onions)
- 2 tablespoons of pine nuts
- Salt and Pepper To Taste

DIRECTIONS

1. Remove the stalks and the first hardest leaves from the fennel.
2. After that, wash them very well and halve lengthwise.
3. Bring salted water to a boil and dip the fennel in it, which you will cook for about 30 minutes.
4. As soon as the fennels are cooked, drain and let them cool.

5. In the meantime, peel the lime (also removing the white skin) and slice them thinly.
6. To prepare the sauce, mix the lime juice with a pinch of salt, plenty of pepper (preferably freshly ground), curry and oil.
7. Beat the ingredients well with a fork until emulsified.
8. Finely slice the shallots or onions.
9. Cut the fennel into strips and put them in a serving salad bowl, sprinkle with the prepared sauce and mix carefully.
10. Decorate the salad with the orange slices and the pine nuts, and then serve.

Orange chickpeas and fennel salad

PREPARATION TIME: 20 minutes

CALORIES: 172

INGREDIENTS FOR 4 SERVINGS

- 2 fennel
- 2 oranges
- 300 grams of cooked chickpeas
- Olive oil to taste
- Salt and pepper to taste

DIRECTIONS

1. Remove the inner part and the harder outer leaves of the fennel. Wash it and cut it into thin slices.
2. Peel the oranges and keep only the pulp. Wash the orange pulp, remove the white filaments and then cut it into cubes.
3. Put the fennel in the bottom of the plates and then put the oranges.
4. Season them with oil, salt and pepper.
5. Finally, put the chickpeas over the fennel and serve.

Cucumber soy yogurt salad

PREPARATION TIME: 10 minutes
CALORIES: 52

INGREDIENTS FOR 4 SERVINGS

- 2 pots of soy yogurt
- 2 cucumbers
- 1 lemon
- 1 sprig of chopped parsley
- Salt and pepper to taste
- Olive oil to taste

DIRECTIONS

1. Wash the cucumbers, cut them into rings and then put them in a salad bowl.
2. In a bowl, put the yogurt and the filtered lemon juice.
3. Add salt, pepper and chopped parsley.
4. Mix well until you get a smooth sauce.
5. Put the yogurt sauce in the salad bowl, mix to flavour well and serve.

Lettuce and cauliflower salad with tofu

PREPARATION TIME: 10 minutes
REST TIME: 15 minutes
CALORIES: 210

INGREDIENTS FOR 4 SERVINGS

- A head of lettuce
- A small cauliflower
- 2 cucumbers
- A bunch of radishes
- 150 grams of tofu cheese
- 1/2 teaspoon of baking soda
- One lemon
- 1 tablespoon of mustard
- sale to taste

DIRECTIONS

1. Prepare all the vegetables well.
2. Remove the oldest leaves from the salad keeping the innermost part, remove the leaves and soak for half an hour in cold water and baking soda.
3. Scrape the cucumbers well without removing the peel, wash them and make small incisions lengthwise.
4. Then slice them not too thinly, sprinkle them with fine salt and put them to make water between two inclined plates.

5. The leaves of the lower part then cut them into slices.

6. Divide the cauliflower into florets and put this in cold water with baking soda.

7. Then after half an hour, drain them and try to bake them into slices.

8. Make regular cubes with the tofu cheese.

9. In a bowl prepare the dressing; put a little lemon juice, more or less to taste and the mustard.

10. Mix well with the help of a fork.

11. On a serving dish first put the well-dried lettuce leaves, the slices of cabbage, then a well-dried slice of cucumber and one of radish, so that the colours alternate, in the centre the cubes of tofu cheese.

12. Serve the sauce separately.

Belgian endive salad with orange

PREPARATION TIME: 10 minutes
COOKING TIME: 25 minutes
CALORIES: 160

INGREDIENTS FOR 4 SERVINGS

- 1 kilo of Belgian endive
- 2 oranges
- 3 tablespoons of oil
- 100 grams of peeled almonds
- Salt and pepper to taste

DIRECTIONS

1. Remove the salad heads from the outer leaves and wash them gently.
2. Bring abundant salted water to a boil in a saucepan.
3. Immerse the tufts in boiling water and cook for 25 minutes, then drain and let them cool.
4. Squeeze the oranges, filter the juice, add the oil and season with salt and pepper.
5. Finely chop the almonds.
6. Arrange the salad on a serving plate, sprinkle it with the preparation juice and sprinkle with the chopped almonds.

Brussels salad

PREPARATION TIME: 20 minutes
CALORIES: 200

INGREDIENTS FOR 4 SERVINGS

- 750 grams of Belgian endive
- 2 apples
- Half a grapefruit
- Half an orange
- Salt and Pepper To Taste
- 2 tablespoons of walnut oil
- 1 tablespoon of peanut oil
- a spoonful of sultanas
- A few walnut kernels

DIRECTIONS

1. Clean the endive salad by removing the hardest and most damaged outer leaves and the core, then wash it thoroughly, dry it gently.
2. Now, cut it into strips.
3. Peel the apples, cut into four parts, remove the central part with the seeds and cut into thin slices.
4. Squeeze half a grapefruit and half an orange into a cup, mixing the two juices together.
5. Add the salt, pepper, and the two types of oil and beat with a fork until the ingredients are well emulsified.

6. Put the endive and apples in a salad bowl and season with the prepared sauce.

7. In the meantime, you have soaked the sultanas in warm water. Dry them and use them, together with the chopped walnut kernels.

8. Decorate the salad with walnuts and serve immediately.

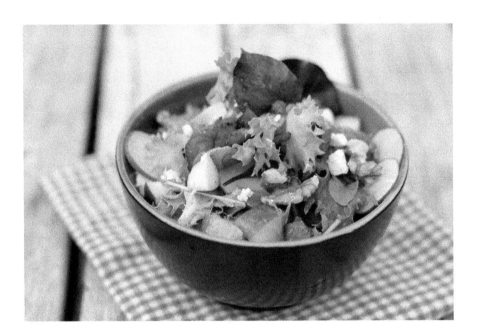

Alsatian salad

PREPARATION TIME: 15 minutes
SOAKING TIME: 2 hours for juniper berries
CALORIES: 200

INGREDIENTS FOR 4 SERVINGS

- A few juniper berries
- 250 grams of sauerkraut in brine
- 150 grams of champignons mushrooms
- The juice of one lemon
- 3 carrots
- 3 onions
- a garlic clove
- A sprig of parsley
- 3 tablespoons of olive oil
- Salt and pepper to taste

DIRECTIONS

1. Soak the juniper berries for 3 hours in a little water to soften them.

2. When the time comes, start preparing the salad.

3. Pass the sauerkraut under running water, and then drain well. Clean the mushrooms, removing all traces of earth, wash them thoroughly and dry them immediately.

4. Then, cut them into slices and sprinkle them with lemon juice to prevent them from blackening.

5. Scrape the carrots or peel them with a sharp knife and grate them with the special tool.

6. Peel the onions and slice them into thin rings.

7. Peel the garlic too and chop finely.

8. At this point, arrange the sauerkraut in the middle of a round serving plate.

9. Drain the juniper berries from the water and sprinkle the mushrooms on the sauerkraut and around them put the grated carrots.

10. Sprinkle the salad with garlic, onion slices and chopped parsley.

11. Add salt and plenty of pepper, better if freshly ground and sprinkle with oil.

12. Bring the salad to the table and mix it just before serving.

Onions and bell peppers salad

PREPARATION TIME: 10 minutes
CALORIES: 178

INGREDIENTS FOR 4 SERVINGS

- 2 large white onions
- A juicy orange
- 1 large green bell pepper
- 100 grams of black olives
- 1 tablespoon of mustard
- the juice of half a lemon
- Olive oil to taste
- 1/2 teaspoon of vegan brown sugar
- Salt pepper to taste

DIRECTIONS

1. Prepare this salad by peeling two white onions and cutting them into thin rings.
2. Take the orange; remove the peel and the white skin between the wedge and the wedge, cutting it with a very sharp knife.
3. Clean the green bell peppers from the seeds and filaments and cut into thin strips.
4. Put all the ingredients in a bowl and add the pitted black olives.
5. Season with an emulsion made with a spoonful of mustard the juice of half a lemon, oil, salt, pepper and half a teaspoon of sugar.
6. Mix well and serve the salad.

Mushrooms and green olives salad

PREPARATION TIME: 10 minutes
CALORIES: 280

INGREDIENTS FOR 4 SERVINGS

- 250 grams of homemade in oil mushrooms
- 200 grams of green olives
- 2 boiled potatoes
- 2 tomatoes
- A stalk of celery
- A meal of salted capers
- 1 teaspoon of mustard
- the juice of one lemon
- a handful of parsley and fresh mint (facultative)
- Olive oil to taste
- salt pepper to taste

DIRECTIONS

1. Drain the mushrooms well.
2. Wash the celery and take the white inside.
3. Cube celery.
4. Put the mushrooms in a salad bowl, the green olives without the stone, the celery cut into cubes, the fresh tomatoes, washed and seeded, the capers washed and cleaned of salt and the two sliced boiled potatoes.

5. Separately dissolve a teaspoon of mustard, lemon juice, oil, salt and abundant pepper and emulsify everything.

6. Then pour over the salad and let it rest for a while, turning every now and then.

7. You can sprinkle with chopped fresh mint and parsley if you want.

Country salad

PREPARATION TIME: 15 minutes
COOKING TIME: 30 minutes
CALORIES: 204

INGREDIENTS FOR 4 SERVINGS

- 400 grams of potatoes
- 3 ripe tomatoes
- A couple of basil leaves
- 1 tablespoon of olive oil
- 1 tablespoon of apple cider vinegar
- Salt and pepper to taste

DIRECTIONS

1. Boil the potatoes directly with the peel.
2. Then drain, peel and cut them still hot into rather large pieces.
3. Boil and peel the tomatoes too.
4. Remove the seeds, drain them and finely chop the pulp collecting it in a bowl.
5. Wash and chop the basil leaves.
6. Add the chopped basil, mix well then add first the vinegar, then the salt, the pepper and finally the oil, beat with a fork, then pour the sauce over the potatoes.
7. Combine all ingredients very well and serve.

Green beans potatoes and tofu salad

PREPARATION TIME: 10 minutes
COOKING TIME: 35 minutes
REST TIME: 1 hour (at least) in the fridge
CALORIES: 252

INGREDIENTS FOR 4 SERVINGS

- 5 potatoes

- 100 grams of green beans

- 150 grams of tofu

- 4/5 Gherkins

- 1 teaspoon of mustard

- Olive oil, salt and pepper to taste

DIRECTIONS

1. Boil the potatoes and green beans separately.

2. After boiling them, peel the potatoes.

3. Cut the potatoes into small pieces and put them in a salad bowl.

4. Cut the green beans into small pieces as well..

5. Cut the tofu into cubes.

6. Now add the green beans to the potatoes and the diced tofu.

7. Season with mustard, oil, salt, pepper.

8. Mix everything well.

9. Cut the gherkins into a flower put it all around the salad.

10. Keep the salad in the refrigerator for at least one hour, then serve.

Avocado salad

PREPARATION TIME: 10 minutes
CALORIES: 290

INGREDIENTS FOR 4 SERVINGS

- 1 avocado
- A bunch of basil
- A bunch of parsley
- 1 small onion or 2 fresh spring onions
- 50 grams of hazelnuts
- 40 grams of walnut kernels
- 250 grams of tofu
- Half a teaspoon of oregano powder
- Salt, pepper, paprika to taste
- some stuffed olives to decorate (facultative)

DIRECTIONS

1. Open the avocado in half lengthwise and remove the core.
2. Then carefully peel off the peel and reduce the pulp into small pieces.
3. Set the avocado pulp aside, while you prepare the other ingredients.
4. Finely chop the basil, parsley, and onion, or spring onions. Separately chop the hazelnuts and walnuts.
5. Put the tofu in a bowl and add the aromatic herbs, the onion, the walnuts and the chopped hazelnuts, mixing well, then add the oregano, salt, pepper in abundance, preferably freshly ground and a good pinch of paprika.
6. Mix again.

7. Then, add the pieces of avocado and stir again gently.

8. Transfer this avocado and tofu salad to a serving bowl and decorate with the stuffed olives. Served chilled.

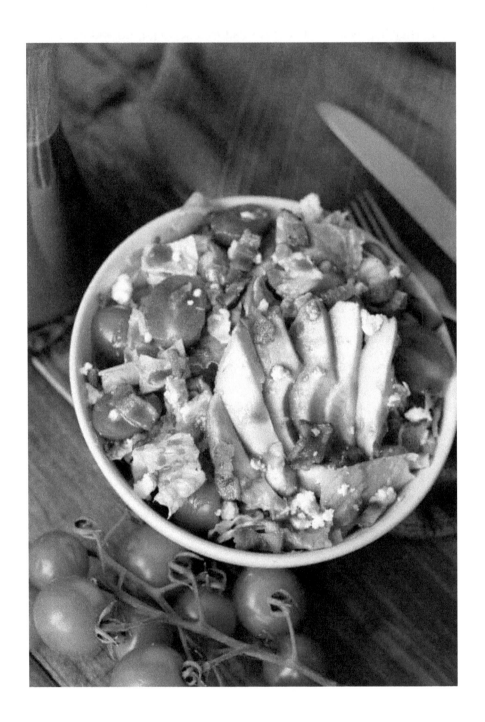

Red cabbage and hazelnuts salad

PREPARATION TIME: 10 minutes
CALORIES: 185

INGREDIENTS FOR 4 SERVINGS

- ½ red cabbage
- The juice of one lemon
- 1 bunch of radishes
- 2 small turnips
- 100 grams of chopped hazelnuts
- 1 teaspoon of mustard
- 3 tablespoons of olive oil
- 1 tablespoon of chopped parsley
- Salt and pepper to taste

DIRECTIONS

1. Remove the hardest leaves from the cabbage.
2. Cut them and wash them thoroughly.
3. Cut them into thin strips, put in a serving salad bowl, and add the salt and the juice of half a lemon.
4. Wash the radishes thoroughly, remove the leaves and cut them into rather small wedges, peel the turnips and grate them in the salad bowl containing the cabbage.
5. Add the radishes too.

6. For the preparation of the sauce, put the mustard in a small bowl and dilute it with the remaining juice of half a lemon and the oil, add the salt, pepper and chopped parsley and mix everything with a fork to emulsify well.

7. Pour the sauce into the salad bowl and mix well. Sprinkle the salad with chopped hazelnuts, and then serve.

Green beans onions and almond cheese

PREPARATION TIME: 10 minutes
COOKING TIME: 30 minutes
CALORIES: 230

INGREDIENTS FOR 4 SERVINGS

- 400 grams of green beans
- 200 grams of spring onions.
- 150 grams of almond homemade cheese (see basic recipe)
- A spoonful of capers
- The juice of one lemon
- Olive oil, salt and pepper to taste

DIRECTIONS

1. After having thoroughly cleaned them, boil the green beans in salted water.
2. Green beans must be very tender and without string.
3. Once cooked, drain them carefully and pour them into a salad bowl.
4. Cook the onions too, these too must be new and small, drain and add them to the green beans.
5. Cut the almond cheese into small cubes.
6. Wash the capers well, which must be those in salt.
7. Now mix all the ingredients well in a bowl.
8. Separately mix olive oil, lemon juice, salt and pepper.
9. Now you can dress the salad with this emulsion.
10. Serve immediately.

Vegetable salad with mayonnaise

PREPARATION TIME: 10 minutes
COOKING TIME: 30 minutes
REST TIME: 1 hour (at least) in the fridge
CALORIES: 360

INGREDIENTS FOR 4 SERVINGS

- 250 grams of green beans
- 250 grams of potatoes
- 250 grams of carrots
- 250 grams of peas
- Plant based mayonnaise (see basic recipe)

DIRECTIONS

1. Wash the potatoes well, peel them and cut them into small cubes.
2. Clean the green beans well by removing the threads, and cut them into small pieces.
3. Wash the carrots too peel them and cut them into cubes like potatoes.
4. Bring salted water to a boil and cook the vegetables, when they are almost cooked add the peas and bring to final cooking.
5. When they are cooked, drain and let them cool. Now put them in a large container and add the mayonnaise, mixing well so that the vegetables are all seasoned.
6. Then put it in a glass dish and put it in the refrigerator for at least an hour before serving.

Summer salad with soy yogurt

PREPARATION TIME: 10 minutes
COOKING TIME: 20 minutes
REST TIME: 1 hour for eggplants, 1 hour (at least) in the fridge for the salad
CALORIES: 160

INGREDIENTS FOR 4 SERVINGS

- 2 bell yellow peppers
- 2 eggplants
- 2 garlic cloves
- A cup of soy yogurt
- The juice of half a lemon
- Olive oil to taste
- 1 pinch of black pepper
- Salt to taste

DIRECTIONS

1. Cut the eggplants into slices then sprinkle them with salt to make them water leaving them with a weight on them for about 1 hour.

2. Wash them, dry them then place them on a grill together with the two bell peppers, cleaned and emptied of seeds, all sprinkled with olive oil.

3. When they are cooked peel both the eggplants and the bell peppers and finely chop both.

4. Put them in a salad bowl; add a cup of soy yogurt, salt, black pepper, two cloves, and minced garlic.

5. Season with oil and the juice of half a lemon.

6. Mix gently and refrigerate at least 1 hour before serving.

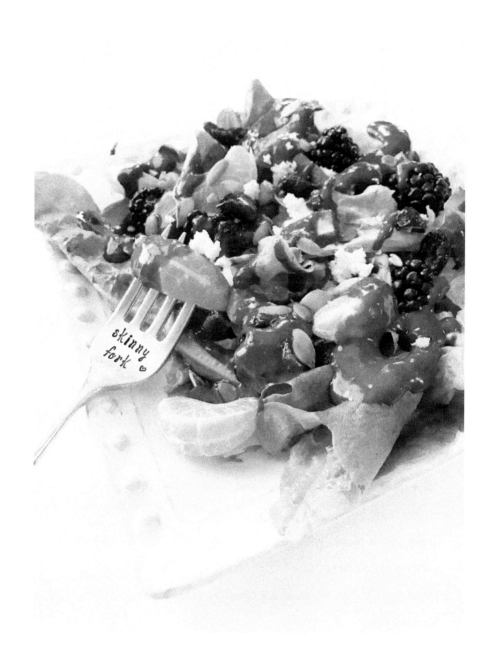

Escarole citrus salad

PREPARATION TIME: 10 minutes
COOKING TIME: 15 minutes
REST TIME: 20 minutes
CALORIES: 110

INGREDIENTS FOR 4 SERVINGS

- A large head of escarole
- 3 spring onions
- 1 celery
- 3 oranges
- 1 lemon
- 2 tablespoons of mustard,
- 1 pinch of baking soda.

DIRECTIONS

1. Take the escarole, clean it well and remove the outer leaves using the whiter part.
2. Break up the leaves with your hands then soak them for half an hour in water and baking soda.
3. Clean two spring onions, braise them into thin slices.
4. Soak them in fresh water.
5. Take the innermost and tender ribs of the celery leaving the leaves as well and divide them into two pieces.

6. Peel lemon and oranges, cut them into slices and clean them well from the skin and seeds.

7. Squeeze half an orange and place it in the salad bowl with a few drops of lemon juice and mustard.

8. Add the well-drained and dried vegetables turning so that they take the sauce well.

9. Garnish the salad with the slices of orange, lemon and celery ribs with the leaves.

10. Place your salad in the fridge.

11. You can serve your salad after 20 minutes fridge rest.

Grand duke Salad

PREPARATION TIME: 10 minutes
COOKING TIME: 25 minutes
REST TIME: 15 minutes
CALORIES: 472

INGREDIENTS FOR 4 SERVINGS

- 1 yellow bell pepper
- 2 zucchini
- One and a half glasses of water
- ½ teaspoon of Tabasco
- Half a lemon
- 100 grams of sultanas
- 200 grams of cooked brown rice
- Olive oil, salt, pepper to taste

DIRECTIONS

1. Wash the bell pepper then put it in the oven to cook for 20 minutes.
2. Once cooked, remove it and skin you will see that the skin comes off easily, clean it from the seeds and cut it into strips.
3. In the meantime, cook the brown rice and drain it al dente, pass it quickly under cold water and put it in a salad bowl.
4. Wash and boil the zucchini for a few minutes.
5. Put the raisins in the water after washing them and finely chop them with the crescent.

6. Add the sliced zucchini to the rice and season the sliced pepper with Tabasco, the raisins removed from the water and mix well.
7. Season with salt, pepper, and a few drops of lemon.
8. You can add a few slices of tomato and diced tofu cheese.
9. Put in the refrigerator for half an hour before serving.

Asparagus and hazelnuts salad

PREPARATION TIME: 10 minutes
COOKING TIME: 10 minutes
CALORIES: 92

INGREDIENTS FOR 4 SERVINGS

- 500 grams of asparagus

- 40 grams of chopped hazelnut

- 1 lemon

- Olive oil to taste

- Salt and pepper to taste

DIRECTIONS

1. Remove the final part of the asparagus, wash them and then cut them into chunks.

2. Heat a tablespoon of olive oil in a pan and as soon as it is hot, sauté the asparagus. Season with salt, pepper, and cook for 10 minutes.

3. In a bowl put the filtered lemon juice, a tablespoon of olive oil, salt and pepper and mix.

4. Now put the asparagus on a serving dish and season with the emulsion.

5. Sprinkle with the chopped hazelnuts and serve.

Stuffed mushrooms turnips

PREPARATION TIME: 10 minutes
COOKING TIME: 60 minutes
CALORIES: 196

INGREDIENTS FOR 4 SERVINGS

- 8 turnips of the same size
- 250 grams of champignons mushrooms
- A clove of garlic, two tablespoons of chopped parsley
- A tablespoon of oil
- 30 grams of soy butter
- 150 grams of grated tofu
- Salt and Pepper To Taste
- homemade vegetable broth (see basic recipe)

DIRECTIONS

1. Peel the turnips, wash and dry them well with a kitchen towel.
2. With a sharp knife cut each turnip about two thirds of the way, removing a cap from the top, which you will keep aside.
3. Then, with the help of a teaspoon, hollow out the turnips entirely to create trays.
4. In doing this last operation, take care not to damage the walls.
5. Sprinkle the inside of the turnips with a pinch of salt.
6. Clean the champignons, scraping them with a small knife, especially on the part of the stalk where the earth is more tenacious.

7. Wash them very carefully and chop them, together with the pulp extracted from the turnips.
8. Chop the garlic too and add it to the other ingredients.
9. Finally add the parsley and mix well.
10. Heat the oil and 10 grams of soy butter in a pan, add the prepared mixture and fry over moderate heat for about 2 minutes.
11. Remove the mince from the heat, transfer it to a bowl and add the grated tofu, salt and pepper.
12. Mix thoroughly.
13. Fill the turnips with the prepared filling and place the cap removed at the beginning on top.
14. Butter one of the turnips, place the stuffed turnips on top and pour a glass of broth into the bowl. Place the pan in the oven and let the turnips cook for 1 hour, adding more broth if the cooking juices tend to dry out too much.
15. Remove from the oven and serve hot, in the same cooking container.

Cream of cucumbers

PREPARATION TIME: 10 minutes
REST TIME: 60 minutes
CALORIES: 135

INGREDIENTS FOR 4 SERVINGS

- 4 pots of soy yogurt
- 1 cucumber
- 500 ml of soymilk
- The juice of half a lemon
- 1 onion
- a garlic clove
- Salt, pepper and vegan brown sugar to taste
- 1 glass of apple cider vinegar
- a sprig of parsley

DIRECTIONS

1. Put the soy yogurt in a bowl together with the soymilk and beat with a whisk.
2. Then, slowly pour in the vinegar and lemon juice.
3. Add the grated onion, the crushed garlic with a little salt, a pinch of pepper and a pinch of sugar.
4. Wash the cucumber well, dry it, and cut a few slices to keep for the garnish.
5. Now, grate the remainder, incorporating it into the prepared mixture.

6. Mix well.

7. Let the cream cool for 1 hour in the refrigerator and serve it garnished with parsley leaves and cucumber slices.

Basil zucchini

PREPARATION TIME: 10 minutes
REST TIME: 60 minutes
CALORIES: 195

INGREDIENTS FOR 4 SERVINGS

- 4 zucchini
- 100 grams of walnut kernels
- 50 grams of pine nuts
- The juice of one lemon
- Olive oil to taste
- Salt and Pepper to taste
- A few basil leaves

DIRECTIONS

1. Wash the zucchini well, they must be very fresh and still with a light fluff.
2. Then slice them very thin.
3. Put zucchini slices in a large bowl and season with abundant oil, salt, pepper and the juice of a lemon.
4. Let it rest for about an hour, making sure to turn them every now and then to soak them well with the sauce.
5. Now, prepare the walnut kernels without the brown skin and pine nuts, chop them carefully with the half moon, then add a little basil, chop, and chop this too.

6. Pour everything on the zucchini.

7. You can serve your zucchini with basil

Zucchini with rice sauce

PREPARATION TIME: 10 minutes
REST TIME: 50 minutes
CALORIES: 285

INGREDIENTS FOR 4/6 SERVINGS

- 8 zucchini
- 150 grams of brown rice
- 1 onion
- 2 tablespoons of soy cream
- 4 tablespoons of homemade tomato sauce
- Olive oil, salt and pepper to taste

DIRECTIONS

1. Clean the zucchini well. Then cut them in half lengthwise and empty the pulp.
2. Blanch them for a few minutes in salted water then drain and set aside.
3. In the meantime, cook the brown rice, which must remain al dente then season it with a few tablespoons of fresh tomato sauce and soy cream.
4. Now chop an onion, which you will add to the soy cream and rice, adjusting with salt and pepper.
5. Beat the mixture well then pour it into a pan with a little oil and scramble it with a fork so that it is creamy.
6. Fill the zucchini with this rice sauce.
7. Place them in a baking pan where you have put some tomato sauce.
8. Put in the oven at 200ºC for about 15 minutes.
9. Serve still hot.

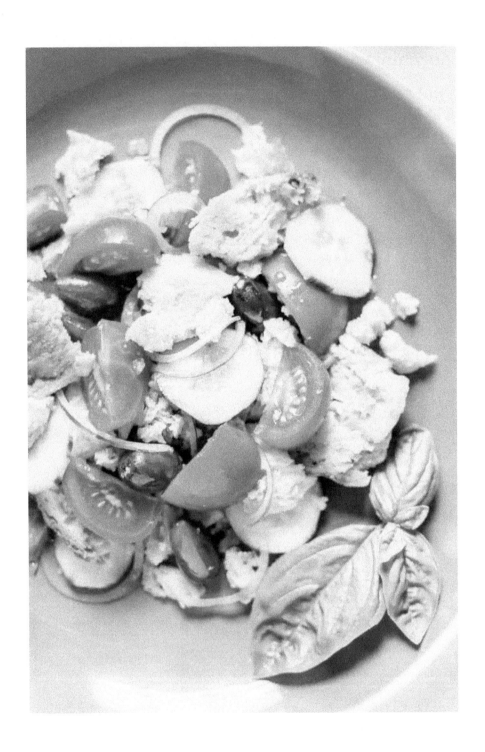

Sweet & Sour vegetables

PREPARATION TIME: 15 minutes
COOKING TIME: 30 minutes
CALORIES: 211

INGREDIENTS FOR 4/6 SERVINGS

- 4 zucchini

- 4 carrots

- 3 ribs of celery

- 4 artichokes

- 1 large eggplant

- Half of a small cauliflower

- 250 grams of cultivated mushrooms

- 12 spring onions

- the juice of one lemon

- A bunch of parsley

- The stalk of a fennel with the leaves attached

- 2 tablespoons of coriander grains two bay leaves

- Pepper in grains, salt to taste

- ½ glass of oil

- 500 ml of apple cider vinegar

- 2 tablespoons of tomato paste

DIRECTIONS

1. Prepare all the vegetables as follows. after washing those that require it, trim the zucchini, scrape the carrots and slice the two ingredients into slices.
2. Then, clean the celery ribs by removing the filaments and cut them into small pieces.
3. Free the artichokes from the hardest outer leaves, stems, thorns and any central hay and divide them into quarters or wedges, according to their size.
4. Remove the stalk from the eggplant and cut into cubes, without peeling.
5. Remove the cauliflower leaves and cut it into florets, scrape the mushrooms with a small knife and leave them whole.
6. Leave the onions completely too.
7. Now, put all the vegetables prepared in a large saucepan, sprinkle them with lemon juice to prevent them from blackening, then add the parsley and the finely chopped inner part of the fennel, the coriander grains, the bay leaf, a dozen peppercorns salt, oil and apple cider vinegar.
8. Place the saucepan on the heat and let the liquid come to a boil keeping the flame moderate, from this moment lower the heat to a minimum and let the preparation quiver (i.e. keep it at the boiling point) for 20 minutes.
9. After this time, add the tomato paste, diluting them in the cooking liquid, cook gently for another 10 minutes.

10. Then, transfer the vegetables with their sauce to a large serving dish and let them cool completely before bringing them to the table.

Zucchini with mushrooms and parsley

PREPARATION TIME: 15 minutes
COOKING TIME: 20 minutes
CALORIES: 155

INGREDIENTS FOR 5/6 SERVINGS

- 750 grams of zucchini
- A handful of dried mushrooms
- 2 garlic cloves
- a sprig of parsley
- 4 tablespoons of oil
- Salt and ground black pepper to taste
- 3 ripe tomatoes

DIRECTIONS

1. Wash the zucchini, trim them and cut them into chunks.
2. Meanwhile, soak the dried mushrooms in hot water to revive them.
3. Prepare a mince with the garlic and parsley.
4. Place it in a large pan with the oil, brown it, and then add the zucchini.
5. Leave it all to flavour for a few minutes, stirring often.
6. Season with salt and pepper.
7. Then, add the mushrooms well squeezed out of their water and wash them.
8. Add the clean tomatoes too, after have removing the peel and seeds.

9. Stir again to mix the ingredients, cover the pan and finish cooking for 10/15 minutes.

10. You can serve both hot and cold.

Marinated zucchini

PREPARATION TIME: 10 minutes
COOKING TIME: 10 minutes
REST TIME: 5/6 hours
CALORIES: 90

INGREDIENTS FOR 4/6 SERVINGS

- 1 kilo of zucchini
- 1 glass of oil
- 1 large glass of vinegar
- 4 cloves of garlic
- 2 bay leaves
- 1 sprig of sage
- 1 sprig of thyme
- 1 sprig of rosemary
- Salt and Pepper To Taste
- a handful of basil

DIRECTIONS

1. Wash the zucchini, dry them and cut them into thin slices of a coin.
2. Then, fry them in the oil that you have made to smoke in the iron pan.
3. Meanwhile, separately, boil the vinegar with bay leaves, sage, and rosemary (tied in a bunch with colourless yarn) when the liquid has reduced by a third.
4. Add salt and pepper and keep warm.

—

5. As the zucchini are ready, lay them in layers in a bowl and season each layer with salt, pepper, basil, slices of garlic and two or three tablespoons of aromatic vinegar.

6. Cover the bowl and keep it in the refrigerator for 5/6 hours before serving.

Baked zucchini with béchamel

PREPARATION TIME: 10 minutes
COOKING TIME: 20 minutes
CALORIES: 194

INGREDIENTS FOR 4 SERVINGS

- 4 large and long zucchini
- 30 grams of soy butter
- 2 tablespoons of grated tofu
- A cup of plant based béchamel (see basic recipe)
- 2 tablespoons of wholemeal breadcrumbs
- Half a glass of soymilk cream
- Salt and pepper to taste

DIRECTIONS

1. Peel and cut the zucchini in half.
2. Wash them and cook them slightly in boiling salted water.
3. When they are blanched, drain and dry them.
4. In a separate bowl, add the soymilk cream, the béchamel, the tofu, and the breadcrumbs.
5. Add the soy butter too and season with salt, pepper.
6. Mix all the ingredients well, then put the zucchini in a buttered pan, cover them with the prepared filling and sprinkle with the pan.
7. Put in the oven to brown for about 15 minutes at 180ºC.
8. Serve zucchini still hot.

Cabbage rolls

PREPARATION TIME: 10 minutes
COOKING TIME: 20 minutes

CALORIES: 255

INGREDIENTS FOR 4 SERVINGS

- A large cabbage
- 300 grams of mushrooms
- A cup plant based of béchamel (see basic recipe)
- Wholemeal breadcrumbs to taste
- 2 cups of homemade tomato sauce
- Olive oil to taste
- Salt and pepper to taste

DIRECTIONS

1. Clean mushrooms by removing any remaining soil.
2. Wash very well cabbage leaves.
3. Put the mushrooms in a bowl, add béchamel and mix well. Add a little of breadcrumbs too, if the mixture is too soft.
4. Then, boil the well-washed cabbage leaves, remove them from the water with a scoop with holes and place them on a cloth so that they dry.
5. Now put the filling and wrap the leaves, fixing them with a toothpick. Put them on the fire with a little oil and the ready-made tomato sauce, add salt and pepper, and cook slowly for a quarter of an hour.
6. Serve the rolls warm.

Cabbage and potato soup

PREPARATION TIME: 10 minutes

COOKING TIME: 55 minutes
CALORIES: 235

INGREDIENTS FOR 6 SERVINGS

- A small savoy cabbage
- 4 potatoes
- 4 carrots
- Vinegar to taste
- 2 onions
- 2 cloves
- 2 ribs of celery
- a bunch of aromatic herbs (thyme, parsley, bay leaf)
- coarse salt to taste
- peppercorns to taste

DIRECTIONS

1. Clean the cabbage by removing the core and the first outer leaves.
2. Then, immerse it repeatedly in water acidulated with vinegar (this procedure will help you eliminate any bacteria).
3. Then place it on the fire in a large saucepan containing cold water and cook for 10 minutes, calculating the time from the moment the water boils.
4. After the indicated time, drain it and cut it into eight wedges.

5. Prepare the other vegetables. Peel and wash the potatoes, scrape the carrots, remove the celery from the leaves and cut it into two or three pieces, peel the onions and stick them with the cloves.

6. Put the cabbage back into the saucepan you used previously in which you will have poured about two litres of cold water and add the prepared vegetables.

7. Complete with the herbs, a good handful of coarse salt and a few peppercorns and cook the soup for about 45 minutes in a covered container and over medium heat.

8. After cooking, remove the casserole with a slotted spoon, first the celery, the aromatic bunch, and the onions, which you will remove, then all the other vegetables that you will put in a heated tureen.

9. Pour the cooking broth over the vegetables and serve immediately, hot.

Leeks soup

PREPARATION TIME: 20 minutes
COOKING TIME: 10 minutes
CALORIES: 142

INGREDIENTS FOR 4 SERVINGS

- 3 large leeks
- A litre of soymilk
- Salt and Pepper To Taste
- 1 glass of soymilk cream
- a sprig of parsley

DIRECTIONS

1. Clean the leeks by removing the inner part and the two outer leaves and about a third of the green part.
2. Then, cut the remaining green part in a cross, reaching the white, and spread out the four edges.
3. Now, immerse each leek, upside down in a large container full of water, pressing the open leaves on the bottom, in order to eliminate any residue of earth.
4. Once this has been done, divide each leek into large pieces, peel and wash the potatoes, then cut them into pieces as well.
5. Pour the soymilk into a saucepan, add an equal amount of water and bring to a boil. Immerse the vegetables in the boiling liquid, add salt and cook for 20 minutes over low heat.

6. After this time, pass everything in vegetable mill, collecting the resulting mixture in a bowl.
7. Now pour the soup into a tureen, sprinkle it with the chervil or parsley, finely chopped.
8. You can serve it both hot and lukewarm.

Leeks and onions croquettes

PREPARATION TIME: 20 minutes
COOKING TIME: 30 minutes
CALORIES: 210

INGREDIENTS FOR 4 SERVINGS

- 1 kilo of leeks and onions
- Salt and Pepper To Taste
- 150 ml of soymilk cream
- 2 tablespoons of potato starch
- 2 tablespoons of tofu cheese
- A spoonful of whole wheat flakes
- A spoonful of mixed aromatic herbs (parsley, sage, basil, rosemary)
- breadcrumbs to taste
- seed oil to taste

DIRECTIONS

1. Remove the inside and half of the green leaves from the leeks.
2. Peel the onions and cut them in half.
3. Bring salted water to a boil in a saucepan and immerse the vegetables, which you cook for about 30 minutes.
4. Then drain the leeks and onions, pass them through a vegetable mill until they are creamy and collect the mixture in a bowl.

5. In another bowl, put the soymilk cream, the potato starch and add the tofu, the wheat flakes and the chopped aromatic herbs, salt and pepper.
6. Mix carefully and add this mixture to the cream of leeks and onions, mixing again carefully.
7. Let the dough rest for a few minutes, then form oval croquettes with them, which you will pass repeatedly in the breadcrumbs.
8. Smoke abundant soybean oil in the frying pan and dip in a few croquettes at a time, making them well browned on each side. As they are ready, place them on a sheet of absorbent kitchen paper and keep them warm.
9. Serve hot.

Aromatic potato salad

PREPARATION TIME: 20 minutes

COOKING TIME: 20 minutes
CALORIES: 340

INGREDIENTS FOR 4 SERVINGS

- 600 grams of potatoes
- 1 avocado
- 1 tablespoon of chopped pistachios
- 1 tablespoon of sesame seeds
- 6 mint leaves
- 1 sprig of chopped parsley
- 1 tablespoon of apple cider vinegar
- Salt and pepper to taste
- Olive oil to taste

DIRECTIONS

1. Wash the potatoes and then put them to cook for 20 minutes in boiling water and salt.
2. Meanwhile, peel and wash the avocado. Remove the stone and cut it into cubes.
3. Put the avocado in a bowl.
4. Drain the potatoes, pass them under cold water and then peel them.

5. Cut them into cubes and put them in the bowl with the avocado.

6. Season with the vinegar, salt, pepper, and mix.

7. Wash and dry the mint leaves and then place them in the bowl with the potatoes.

8. Sprinkle with chopped parsley and chopped pistachios and serve.

Pineapple and celery salad

PREPARATION TIME: 15 minutes
CALORIES: 200

INGREDIENTS FOR 4 SERVINGS

- 400 grams of peeled pineapple
- 100 grams of rocket
- 4 stalks of celery
- 20 grams of chopped walnuts
- 250 grams of soy yogurt
- 1 sprig of chopped parsley
- Olive oil to taste
- Salt and pepper to taste

DIRECTIONS

1. Wash and dry the rocket.
2. Remove the stalk of celery and remove the lateral filaments. Wash the celery and then cut them into slices.
3. Wash the pineapple pulp, dry it and then cut it into cubes.
4. Put the yogurt in a bowl. Add salt, parsley and pepper and mix well.
5. Put the rocket on the bottom of the salad bowl. Put the celery and pineapple on top.
6. Dress the salad with the yogurt sauce, sprinkle it with the chopped walnuts and serve

Flavoured fennel and leeks

PREPARATION TIME: 10 minutes
COOKING TIME: 30 minutes

CALORIES: 140

INGREDIENTS FOR 4 SERVINGS

- 4 fennel
- 4 leeks
- 2 bay leaves
- 1 tablespoon of coriander seeds
- 1 lemon
- 100 grams of tomato pulp
- Olive oil to taste
- Salt and pepper to taste

DIRECTIONS

1. Remove the beard and the hardest fennel leaves. Wash them and then cut them first into wedges and then into slices.
2. Remove the green part of the leeks, wash them and then cut them into slices.
3. Wash and dry the lemon and then grate the zest.
4. Put two tablespoons of olive oil, lemon zest, and bay leaf and coriander seeds in a pan.
5. Stir, cook for a minute and then add the leeks and fennel.
6. Stir again, sauté them for 4 minutes and then add the tomato pulp.

7. Cover the pan and cook over medium heat for 20 minutes.

8. After 20 minutes, season with salt and pepper, mix and turn off.

9. Put the vegetables on serving plates and serve.

Oven-roasted tomatoes

PREPARATION TIME: 10 minutes

COOKING TIME: 35 minutes
CALORIES: 45

INGREDIENTS FOR 4 SERVINGS

- 500 grams of cherry tomatoes
- 1 sprig of thyme
- 1 sprig of rosemary
- A tablespoon of dried oregano
- 4 sage leaves
- Salt and pepper to taste
- Olive oil to taste

DIRECTIONS

1. Wash and dry the cherry tomatoes and then cut them in half.
2. Take a baking sheet and line it with parchment paper.
3. Put the cherry tomatoes inside.
4. Wash and dry the thyme, rosemary and sage and then chop them.
5. Sprinkle the tomatoes with oregano and other aromatic herbs.
6. Season with oil, salt, pepper, and cook in the oven at 180 ° C for 35 minutes.
7. Once cooked, take them out of the oven, put them on plates and serve.

Golden zucchini

PREPARATION TIME: 10 minutes
COOKING TIME: 10 minutes
CALORIES: 91

INGREDIENTS FOR 4 SERVINGS

- 2 zucchinis
- 40 grams of oat flour
- 40 ml of soymilk
- Salt and pepper to taste
- Olive oil to taste

DIRECTIONS

1. Wash the zucchinis and then cut them into slices.
2. Put the soymilk in a bowl and the oatmeal in a plate.
3. Put salt and pepper in the bowl with the milk and mix.
4. Now pass the slices of zucchini first in the milk and then in the flour.
5. Heat two tablespoons of oil in a pan and when hot, cook the zucchinis for 4 minutes per side.
6. When they are cooked, place them on two sheets of absorbent paper to absorb excess oil.
7. Now put them on the serving plates and serve.

Onions with mustard sauce

PREPARATION TIME: 15 minutes
COOKING TIME: 40 minutes
CALORIES: 310

INGREDIENTS FOR 4 SERVINGS

- 6 onions
- 400 ml of plant based béchamel
- 2 tablespoons of mustard
- 1 teaspoon of mustard
- Olive oil to taste
- Salt and pepper to taste

DIRECTIONS

1. Remove the cap from the onions, then peel and wash them.
2. Put the onions in a pan with cold water and salt and cook for 30 minutes.
3. Drain the onions and set aside the cooking juices.
4. Put the béchamel in a saucepan and bring to a boil.
5. Turn off, and add the mustard and paprika and mix well.
6. Brush a baking pan with olive oil and put the onions inside.
7. Sprinkle the surface of the onions with the béchamel and put in the oven.
8. Cook at 180°C for 10 minutes.
9. After 10 minutes, take the onions out of the oven; let them cool for 5 minutes.
10. Now put them on the plates and serve.

Gratin onions

PREPARATION TIME: 15 minutes
COOKING TIME: 40 minutes
CALORIES: 110

INGREDIENTS FOR 4 SERVINGS

- 1 kilo of onions
- Wholemeal breadcrumbs to taste
- 100 ml of apple cider vinegar
- Olive oil to taste
- Salt and pepper to taste

DIRECTIONS

1. Remove the onion cap, peel and wash them.
2. Bring a saucepan of water, salt and apple cider vinegar to a boil.
3. As soon as it comes to a boil, cook the onions for 15 minutes.
4. After 15 minutes, drain the onions, let them cool and then cut them in half.
5. Take a baking tray and cover it with parchment paper.
6. Put the onions inside. Season them with oil, salt and pepper.
7. Sprinkle them with breadcrumbs and put them in the oven.
8. Cook at 180 ° C for 20 minutes.
9. After the cooking time, take the onions out of the oven and let them rest for 2 minutes.
10. Now put the onions on the plates and serve.

Pumpkin glazed with soy and sesame

PREPARATION TIME: 15 minutes
COOKING TIME: 20 minutes
CALORIES: 93

INGREDIENTS FOR 4 SERVINGS

- 400 grams of pumpkin already peeled
- 40 grams of vegan whole cane sugar
- 2 tablespoons of soy sauce
- 20 grams of sesame seeds
- Olive oil to taste
- Salt and pepper to taste

DIRECTIONS

1. Put the sesame seeds in a non-stick pan and then let them toast for a couple of minutes.
2. As soon as they are well toasted, turn them off and set aside.
3. Now wash the pumpkin pulp and cut it into cubes.
4. Put the soy sauce and sugar in a pan. Melt the sugar and then add the pumpkin.
5. Sauté for 2-3 minutes and then season with salt and pepper.
6. Add a few tablespoons of water and cook for 15 minutes.
7. After the cooking time, turn off and let cool.
8. Now put the pumpkin on serving plates, sprinkle with sesame seeds and serve.

Pan-fried mushrooms and beans

PREPARATION TIME: 20 minutes
COOKING TIME: 1 hour and 20 minutes
CALORIES: 111

INGREDIENTS FOR 4 SERVINGS

- 300 grams of beans
- 400 grams of mushrooms
- 4 tomatoes
- 1 clove of garlic
- 2 bay leaves
- Olive oil to taste
- Salt and Pepper To Taste.

DIRECTIONS

1. Wash and dry the bay leaf and put it in a pot with the beans.
2. Cover them with cold water, add salt and pepper, and then cook them for 60 minutes.
3. Meanwhile, remove the earthy part of the mushrooms, wash them under running water, dry them and then cut them into slices.
4. Peel and wash the garlic.
5. Wash the tomatoes and cut them into cubes.
6. Heat a drizzle of olive oil in a pan and as soon as it is hot, brown the garlic for a couple of minutes.

7. Add the mushrooms, mix and cook for 3 minutes.

8. Now add the tomatoes, season with salt and pepper and mix. Continue cooking for another 10 minutes, stirring occasionally.

9. After 10 minutes, turn off.

10. As soon as the beans are cooked, drain them and put them, together with a ladle of cooking juices, in the pan with the mushrooms.

11. Turn it back on and cook for another 5 minutes.

12. After 5 minutes, turn off, put on serving plates and serve.

Ratatouille

PREPARATION TIME: 15 minutes
COOKING TIME: 30 minutes
CALORIES: 105

INGREDIENTS FOR 4 SERVINGS

- 1 eggplant
- 1 yellow pepper
- 3 courgettes
- 2 cloves of garlic
- 1 onion
- 1 red pepper
- 3 tomatoes
- 1 sprig of chopped parsley
- Apple cider vinegar to taste
- Olive oil to taste
- Salt and Pepper To Taste.

DIRECTIONS

1. Wash the peppers.
2. Heat a grill and grill the peppers for 15 minutes, turning them on all sides.
3. As soon as they are cooked, put them in a bowl and let them cool. As soon as they are cold, peel them; remove the stalk, seeds and white filaments. Now cut the peppers into strips.
4. Wash the tomatoes and then cut them into cubes.

5. Wash the zucchinis and then cut them into slices.

6. Wash the eggplant and then cut it into cubes.

7. Peel and wash the onion and then cut it into slices.

8. Peel and wash the garlic cloves.

9. Heat two tablespoons of olive oil in a pan and brown the garlic and onion for a couple of minutes.

10. Now add the zucchinis and mix.

11. Now add the eggplant, tomatoes and peppers and mix again.

12. Season with salt, pepper, and cook for 20 minutes.

13. Now blend the vegetables with two tablespoons of apple cider vinegar and then turn off.

14. Sprinkle with chopped parsley and serve.

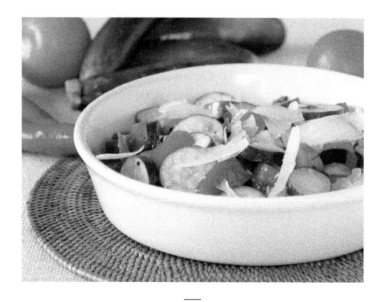

Dessert and fruit recipes

Chocolate and vanilla bread

PREPARATION TIME: 20 minutes
COOKING TIME: 30 minutes
CALORIES: 490

INGREDIENTS FOR 4 SERVINGS

- 130 grams of all wholemeal flour
- 70 grams of vegan brown sugar
- 1 tablespoon of sugar free cocoa powder
- 1 tablespoon of coconut oil
- 1 teaspoon of baking soda
- 1 teaspoon of vanilla extract
- 80 ml of olive oil
- 30 grams of chopped dark vegan chocolate
- 30 grams of chopped almonds

DIRECTIONS

1. Melt the coconut oil in the microwave and then combine with cocoa powder.
2. Add the olive oil too and then blend everything until you get a creamy and homogeneous mixture.
3. Sift the flour into a bowl. Add the baking soda, vanilla extract and brown sugar.
4. Mix everything well with a wooden spoon.

5. When the mixture is homogeneous and blended, add the chopped dark chocolate and the chopped almonds.
6. Take a baking pan and brush it with a little olive oil.
7. Pour the mixture inside and beat gently to level well.
8. Cook at 200ºC for 30 minutes.
9. After 30 minutes check the cooking and if it is still not well done, continue for another 5 minutes.
10. As soon as it is ready, take it out of the oven and let it cool.
11. Turn over into a serving dish, cut into slices and serve.

Chocolate coconut and pistachios bread

PREPARATION TIME: 20 minutes
COOKING TIME: 30 minutes
CALORIES: 490

INGREDIENTS FOR 4 SERVINGS

- 100 grams of all wholemeal flour
- 40 grams of coconut flour
- 60 grams of vegan brown sugar
- 1 tablespoon of sugar free cocoa powder
- 1 tablespoon of coconut oil
- 1 teaspoon of baking soda
- ½ teaspoon of nutmeg
- 1 pinch of vanilla powder
- 80 ml of coconut milk
- 30 grams of chopped dark vegan chocolate
- 40 grams of chopped pistachios

DIRECTIONS

1. Melt the coconut oil in the microwave and then combine with cocoa powder.
2. Add the coconut milk too and then blend everything until you get a creamy and homogeneous mixture.
3. Sift the wholemeal and coconut flour into a bowl. Add the baking soda, vanilla and nutmeg powder and brown sugar.

4. Mix everything well with a wooden spoon.

5. When the mixture is homogeneous and blended, add the chopped dark chocolate and the chopped pistachios.

6. Take a baking pan and brush it with a little olive oil.

7. Pour the mixture inside and beat gently to level well.

8. Cook at 200ºC for 30 minutes.

9. After 30 minutes check the cooking and if it is still not well done, continue for another 5 minutes.

10. As soon as it is ready, take it out of the oven and let it cool.

11. Turn over into a serving dish, cut into slices and serve.

Soy and Apple bread with chocolate

PREPARATION TIME: 20 minutes
COOKING TIME: 30 minutes
CALORIES: 525

INGREDIENTS FOR 4 SERVINGS

- 140 grams of all wholemeal flour
- 1 teaspoon of coconut oil
- 60 grams of vegan brown sugar
- 1 teaspoon of baking soda
- 1 pinch of ginger powder
- 2 small apples
- 100 ml of soy yogurt
- 30 grams of chopped dark vegan chocolate
- 30 grams of chopped pistachios

DIRECTIONS

1. Peel and wash the apples.
2. Wash them and then dry them.
3. Cut them into slices and then transfer them to the blender glass.
4. Melt the coconut oil in the microwave and then add it to the apples.
5. Also add the soy yogurt and then blend everything until you get a creamy and homogeneous mixture.
6. Sift the flour into a bowl. Add the baking soda, ginger powder and sugar.

7. Stir and then add the mixture to the apples, mixing everything with a wooden spoon.

8. When the mixture is homogeneous and blended, add the chopped dark chocolate and the chopped pistachios.

9. Take a baking pan and brush it with a little olive oil.

10. Pour the mixture inside and beat gently to level well.

11. Cook at 200ºC for 30 minutes.

12. After 30 minutes check the cooking and if it is still not well done, continue for another 5 minutes.

13. As soon as it is ready, take it out of the oven and let it cool.

14. Turn over into a serving dish, cut into slices and serve.

Coconut and apple bread

PREPARATION TIME: 20 minutes
COOKING TIME: 30 minutes
CALORIES: 480

INGREDIENTS FOR 4 SERVINGS

- 100 grams of all wholemeal flour

- 40 grams of coconut flour

- 1 teaspoon of coconut oil

- 60 grams of vegan brown sugar

- 1 teaspoon of baking soda

- 1 pinch of nutmeg

- 2 small apples

- 100 ml of soy yogurt

- 30 grams of chopped hazelnuts

DIRECTIONS

1. Peel and wash the apples.

2. Wash them and then dry them.

3. Cut them into slices and then transfer them to the blender glass.

4. Melt the coconut oil in the microwave and then add it to the apples.

5. Also add the soy yogurt and then blend everything until you get a creamy and homogeneous mixture.

6. Sift the flour into a bowl. Add the baking soda, nutmeg and sugar.

7. Stir and then add the mixture to the apples, mixing everything with a wooden spoon.

8. When the mixture is homogeneous and blended, add the chopped hazelnuts.

9. Take a baking pan and brush it with a little olive oil.

10. Pour the mixture inside and beat gently to level well.

11. Cook at 200ºC for 30 minutes.

12. After 30 minutes check the cooking and if it is still not well done, continue for another 5 minutes.

13. As soon as it is ready, take it out of the oven and let it cool.

14. Turn over into a serving dish, cut into slices and serve.

Raspberry and soy bread

PREPARATION TIME: 25 minutes
REST TIME: 2 and 30 minutes hours
COOKING TIME: 25 minutes
CALORIES: 310

INGREDIENTS FOR 4 SERVINGS

- 200 grams of wholemeal flour

- 50 grams of soy flour

- 35 grams of soy butter

- 15 grams of brown vegan sugar

- 12 grams of yeast (based cremor tart)

- 100 ml of soy yogurt

- 60 grams of raspberries already cleaned

- a pinch of salt

DIRECTIONS

1. First, put the two flours, sugar and salt in a bowl.

2. Meanwhile wash raspberries and let dry them.

3. Take half of soy yogurt and add it to the flours.

4. Melt the soy butter and then add it to the rest of the ingredients.

5. Pour the yeast too and start kneading the mixture with your hands.

6. Knead until you get a smooth and homogeneous dough.

7. Add the raspberries and knead a little more.

8. Put the dough to rise covered with a warm cloth and put in a dry and warm place for 2 hours.

9. Grease a rectangular mold and transfer the dough directly into the mold.
10. Let it rest for other 30 minutes.
11. Preheat your oven at 200º C.
12. Place the mold in the oven and let bread cook for 30/35 minutes.
13. Check the cooking and if the raspberry bread is ready remove from the oven.
14. Let cool, cut into slices and serve.

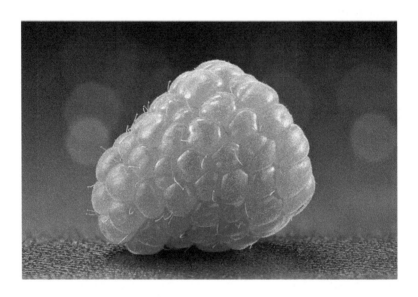

Strawberry ginger bread

PREPARATION TIME: 25 minutes
REST TIME: 2 and 30 minutes hours
COOKING TIME: 25 minutes
CALORIES: 350

INGREDIENTS FOR 4 SERVINGS

- 200 grams of wholemeal flour
- 50 grams of almond flour
- 35 grams of almond butter
- 15 grams of brown vegan sugar
- 12 grams of yeast (based cremor tart)
- 1 teaspoon of ginger powder
- 100 ml of soy yogurt
- 100 grams of strawberries
- a pinch of salt

DIRECTIONS

1. First, put the two flours, ginger powder, sugar and salt in a bowl.
2. Meanwhile wash strawberries, removing the stalk, and let dry them.
3. Take half of soy yogurt and add it to the flours.
4. Melt the almond butter and then add it to the rest of the ingredients.
5. Pour the yeast too and start kneading the mixture with your hands.
6. Knead until you get a smooth and homogeneous dough.
7. Add the strawberries and knead a little more.

8. Put the dough to rise covered with a warm cloth and put in a dry and warm place for 2 hours.

9. Grease a rectangular mold and transfer the dough directly into the mold.

10. Let it rest for other 30 minutes.

11. Preheat your oven at 200º C.

12. Place the mold in the oven and let bread cook for 30/35 minutes.

13. Check the cooking and if the raspberry bread is ready remove from the oven.

14. Let cool, cut into slices and serve.

Cinnamon and vanilla bread

PREPARATION TIME: 15 minutes
REST TIME: 2 hours
COOKING TIME: 35 minutes
CALORIES: 320

INGREDIENTS FOR 6 SERVINGS

- 230 grams of wholemeal flour
- 120 ml of almond milk
- 45 grams of olive oil
- 2 tablespoons of soy yogurt
- 6 grams of natural yeast
- 35 grams of vegan brown sugar
- 1 pinch of salt
- 15 grams of cinnamon powder
- 10 grams of vanilla powder
- 15 grams of stevia powder
- 10 grams of sun flower oil

DIRECTIONS

1. First, put the almond milk and olive oil in a saucepan.
2. Let the almond milk cool for a couple of minutes and then add the yeast.
3. Stir and then let the mixture rest for 10 minutes.
4. Put the brown sugar, a pinch of salt and the soy yogurt in a bowl.

5. Combine these ingredients with an electric mixer and when you have obtained a light and fluffy cream, add the milk and half the wholemeal flour.

6. Stir until the flour is completely incorporated, and then add the rest of the flour.

7. Work the dough at medium speed for 10 minutes.

8. Remove the dough from the bowl, form a ball and put it to rest for 2 hours in another bowl brushed with oil and covered.

9. After the resting time, put the dough on a lightly floured pastry board and roll out the dough trying to make a rectangle more or less 30-40 cm long.

10. Brush the entire surface with sunflower oil.

11. Mix the stevia, vanilla and cinnamon and then distribute it over the entire surface of the dough.

12. Roll the dough on itself and pinch the edge with a fork to seal it.

13. Brush a loaf pan with oil and then put the dough inside, placing the closing part at the bottom.

14. Cover and let rise for another two hours.

15. When this time has passed, place the dough in a baking pan.

16. Cook at 180ºC for 35 minutes.

17. Check the cooking and if not yet cooked continue for another 10 minutes.

18. As soon as it is ready, remove it from the oven cut it into slices and serve the bread with jam to your liking.

Coconut and vanilla bread

PREPARATION TIME: 15 minutes
REST TIME: 2 hours
COOKING TIME: 35 minutes
CALORIES: 320

INGREDIENTS FOR 6 SERVINGS

- 200 grams of wholemeal flour
- 50 grams of coconut flour
- 150 ml of coconut milk
- 45 grams of coconut oil
- 2 tablespoons of soy yogurt
- 6 grams of natural yeast
- 35 grams of vegan brown sugar
- 1 pinch of salt
- 10 grams of vanilla powder
- 10 grams of sun flower oil

DIRECTIONS

1. First, melt the coconut oil in the microwave.
2. Then put the coconut milk and oil in a saucepan.
3. When boiled, let the coconut milk cool for a couple of minutes and then add the yeast.
4. Stir and then let the mixture rest for 10 minutes.
5. Put the brown sugar, a pinch of salt and the soy yogurt in a bowl.
6. Combine these ingredients with an electric mixer and when you have obtained a light and fluffy cream, add the milk and half the wholemeal flour.

7. Now add the two flours.

8. Stir until the two flours is completely incorporated, and then add the rest of the flour.

9. Work the dough at medium speed for 10 minutes.

10. Remove the dough from the bowl, form a ball and put it to rest for 2 hours in another bowl brushed with oil and covered.

11. After the resting time, put the dough on a lightly floured pastry board and roll out the dough trying to make a rectangle more or less 30-40 cm long.

12. Brush the entire surface with sunflower oil.

13. Distribute vanilla powder over the entire surface of the dough.

14. Roll the dough on itself and pinch the edge with a fork to seal it.

15. Brush a loaf pan with oil and then put the dough inside, placing the closing part at the bottom.

16. Cover and let rise for another two hours.

17. When this time has passed, place the dough in a baking pan.

18. Cook at 180ºC for 35 minutes.

19. Check the cooking and if not yet cooked continue for another 10 minutes.

20. As soon as it is ready, remove it from the oven cut it into slices and serve the bread with jam to your liking.

Almond and soy bread

PREPARATION TIME: 15 minutes
COOKING TIME: 30 minutes
CALORIES: 300

INGREDIENTS FOR 6/8 SERVINGS

- 250 grams of wholemeal flour
- 200 grams of corn starch
- 12 grams of natural Baking Powder
- 30 grams of almond flour
- 120 grams of vegan brown sugar
- 1 pinch of salt
- 250 ml of almond milk
- 100 ml of soy yogurt
- 15 ml of vegetable oil
- 15 ml of Honey

DIRECTIONS
1. Start the recipe by beating yogurt with sugar.
2. Beat them until you will reach a thick and foamy compound.
3. Meanwhile, combine the wholemeal flour, almond flour, corn starch, baking powder and salt, in a large bowl and stir.
4. Combine the almond milk, the soy yogurt mix, vegetable oil in a separate small bowl and whisk together.
5. Add the liquid mixture to the dry mixture and stir to just combine.

6. Grease an 8 x 8 baking dish with the rest of the oil.

7. Preheat oven at 190° C.

8. Let bake almond and soy bread at least for 30 minutes.

9. Cook until a toothpick inserted into the centre comes out clean and top has lightly browned.

10. Remove the baking pan from the oven and let cool briefly before serving.

Orange and almond bread

PREPARATION TIME: 15 minutes
COOKING TIME: 30 minutes
CALORIES: 300

INGREDIENTS FOR 6/8 SERVINGS

- 200 grams of wholemeal flour
- 200 grams of almond flour
- 1 orange juice
- 12 grams of natural Baking Powder
- 100 grams of vegan brown sugar
- 1 pinch of salt
- 250 ml of almond milk
- 100 ml of soy yogurt
- 15 ml of vegetable oil
- 15 ml of Honey
- Orange zest (to decorate)

DIRECTIONS

1. Start the recipe by beating yogurt with sugar.
2. Beat them until you will reach a thick and foamy compound.
3. Meanwhile, combine the wholemeal flour, almond flour, baking powder and salt, in a large bowl and stir.
4. Wash and squeeze the orange in order to take the juice.

5. Combine the almond milk, the soy yogurt mix, orange juice, vegetable oil in a separate small bowl and whisk together.

6. Add the liquid mixture to the dry mixture and stir to just combine.

7. Grease an 8 x 8 baking dish with the rest of the oil.

8. Preheat oven at 190° C.

9. Let bake almond and orange y bread at least for 30 minutes.

10. Cook until a toothpick inserted into the centre comes out clean and top has lightly browned.

11. Remove the baking pan from the oven and let cool briefly before serving.

12. Serve bread decorating with orange zest.

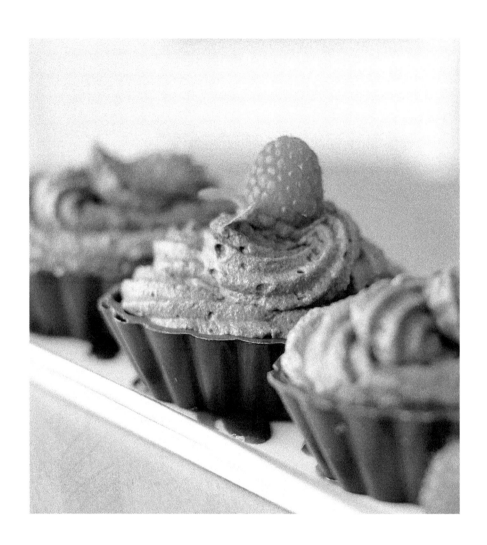

A Plant-Based Diet Cookbook

Lose weight and stay fit with easy and
delicious Plant-Based recipes

Carolyn J. Perez

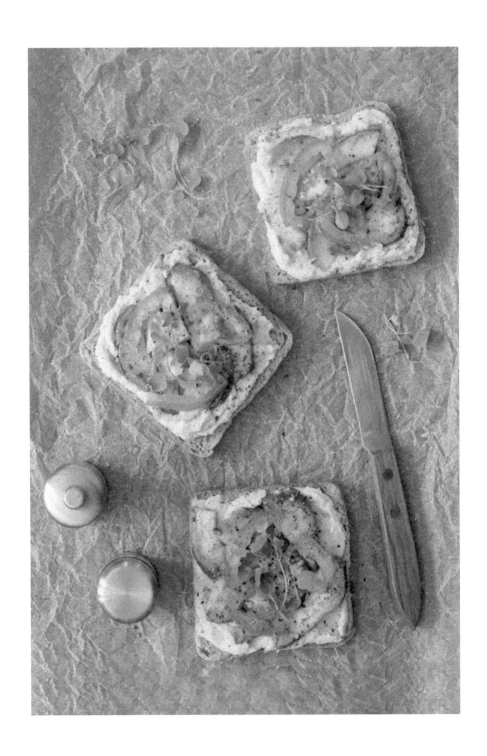

Contents

INTRODUCTION 119

PLANT BASED DIET: WHAT ARE WE TALKING ABOUT? 121

MAIN DIFFERENCES BETWEEN VEGAN AND PLANT BASED DIET
.... 123

Avocado and lime hummus.. 132
Spicy avocado orange hummus.. 134
Fried bread with red lentils and mango humus 136
Raisins coleslaw.. 138
Cannellini beans and olive slices 139
Quinoa pods 141
Spicy cauliflower.. 142
Sweet potato and chicory toast 143
Edamame cream toast.. 145
Veggies Strudel.. 147
Zucchini and ricotta Strudel 149
Zucchini and soy yogurt pie.. 151
Tofu and zucchini plum cake 152
Peas and asparagus plum cake.. 154
Almond cheese asparagus 156
Tofu and figs canapés 158
Eggplant and herbs cream canapés 160
Basil and tofu cream canapés 162
Artichokes and tofu cream canapés 163
Tofu and avocado canapés 165
Soy cheese and cucumber canapés 167
Avocado and rice milk cream 169
Spiced soy avocado.. 170
Avocado chips with paprika mayonnaise 172
PASTA AND CEREALS 174
Wholemeal penne with seitan and hazelnuts...................... 174
Wholemeal spaghetti in red bell pepper sauce................... 176
Vegetarian dim sum.. 178
Wholemeal macaroni with broccoli and basil...................... 181
Potato gnocchi with asparagus and peas............................ 183
Pumpkin gnocchi with soy butter and sage 185
Wholemeal tagliatelle with bean cream 186
Couscous with mushrooms and peas................................... 188
Zucchini noodles with baked tofu....................................... 190

Wholemeal pasta with seitan sauce *192*
Wholemeal penne with broccoli, cauliflower and *194*
almonds *194*
Quinoa with tempeh and vegetables *196*
Quinoa with pumpkin, hazelnuts and coriander *198*
Quinoa tomato and basil *200*
Carrot gnocchi with mushroom sauce *201*
Carrot gnocchi with tomato sauce and capers *203*
Potato gnocchi with asparagus cream *205*
Potato gnocchi with mushrooms and cherry tomatoes *207*
Potato gnocchi with mushrooms and saffron *209*
Potato gnocchi with peppers and cherry tomatoes *211*
Wholemeal pasta salad with tofu, black olives *213*
and cherry tomatoes *213*
Wholemeal penne with pumpkin and onion *215*
Soy noodles with vegetables *217*
Wholemeal spaghetti with saffron and pumpkin *219*
Wholemeal tagliatelle with pumpkin and mushrooms *221*

Introduction

It is a common thought to think that following a diet is necessarily linked to the concept of actual weight loss. However, this is not always the case: following a diet is often directly linked to the foods that we decide to include in our tables daily.

In addition, we do not always choose the best quality ingredients to cook our dishes.

Sometimes we are so rushed and unruly that we forget that we love our bodies. And what better cure than a healthy diet? Following a healthy diet should become more than an imposition or a punishment, but a real lifestyle.

Moreover, this is the Plant-based diet goal: not to impose a restrictive and sometimes impossible diet to follow, but to recreate a diet based on foods of natural origin and above all healthy. Therefore, the plant based represents a real food trend. However, as we will see it is much more than just a fashion trend, but a real lifestyle.

In addition, it is the aim of this text, or rather of this cookbook, to introduce you to the plant based discipline. And we will do it with a few theoretical explanations, just to make you understand what we are talking about and above all how to prepare it: there will be a purely practical part where you will find 50 recipes on the plant based. These recipes will be divided into appetizers, snacks, first and second courses, side dishes and finally a string of plant based desserts.

In the end, you will be spoiled for choice to start following this healthy dietary discipline.

Plant based diet: what are we talking about?

We already mentioned that more than a real weight loss diet the Plant based diet is a food discipline. Food discipline is enjoying great success not only because it is very fashionable, but because it applies such principles that can be perfectly integrated into our daily lives. The plant-based diet is a true approach to life, starting with nutrition: respect for one's health and body, first of all, which is reflected in respect for all forms of life and the planet in general.

As the word itself says, it deals with a food plan based, precisely on what comes from plants. However, simply calling it that way would be too simplistic.

It is a predominantly plant-based diet, but not only. It is not just about consuming vegetables but about taking natural foods: not industrially processed, not treated, and not deriving from the exploitation of resources and animals, preferably zero km.

So it could be a discipline that aims not only at environmental saving but also at the economic one: think about what advantages, in fact, at the level of your pockets you can have if you apply the principle of 0Km and therefore to be able to harvest your vegetables directly from your garden.

Environmental savings do not only mean pollution reduction: the ethical component (present exclusively in the vegan diet, for example) is combined with a strong will to health. This means that the plant based, in addition to not preferring foods that exploit animals, is also based on foods that are especially unprocessed, fresh, healthy, balanced, light, and rich in essential nutrients. In practice, it is a plant-based diet but not vegan / vegetarian, emphasizing the quality and wholesomeness of foods rather than on their moral value, albeit with great attention to sustainability. Such a lifestyle could therefore be of help, not only to our health, but also to create a more sustainable world for future generations.

Main differences between Vegan and Plant based diet

The plant-based diet is often associated with the vegan diet. This is because both plan to include cruelty free foods that do not involve any animal exploitation.

Furthermore, they are associated precisely because they are both predominantly plant-based.

However, there are some pretty obvious differences between these two diets.

First of all, precisely for the reasoning behind the prevalence of plants.

It is well known that even the vegan diet provides a diet based on foods of plant origin: unlike the plant-based diet, however, nothing of animal derivation is allowed, neither direct nor indirect, nor other products - clothing or accessories - which include the exploitation of animals.

No eggs, no milk, no honey, no leather, so to speak, and not only: in its most rigorous meanings, veganism does not even include the use of yeasts, as the bacteria that compose them are indisputably living beings.

A vegan diet can be balanced if the person who leads it knows well the foods and their combinations, the necessary supplements, and their body's reaction to the lack of certain foods.

On the contrary, the Plant-Based diet is on the one hand more relaxed, on the other more stringent.

What does it mean?

This means that it is on the one hand more relaxed because it is plant-based, but not exclusively vegetable: products of animal origin are allowed, in moderate quantities, but under only one condition, namely the excellent quality of the food itself and its certified origin. For example, eggs can be consumed occasionally but only if very fresh, possibly at zero km, from free-range farms where the hens are not exploited but can live outdoors without constraints.

It is also a somewhat more stringent philosophy than veganism precisely for this reason: as long as it is 100% vegetable, the vegan also consumes heavily processed foods, such as industrial fries. Therefore, the vegan can also eat junk foods or snacks. Conversely, plant-based dieters would never admit highly refined foods of this type.

Both dietary approaches are conscious and do not involve the consumption of meat. However, if vegans are driven by ethical reasons, those who follow a plant-based diet also reject everything processed on an industrial level and unhealthy.

A plant-based diet is a diet that aims to eliminate industrially processed foods and, therefore, potentially more harmful to health. It is based on the consumption of fruit and vegetables, whole grains and avoiding (or minimizing) animal products and processed foods. This means that vegan desserts made with refined sugar or bleached flour are also covered.

There is also a substantial difference between the philosophies behind the two diets. As we said in the previous paragraph and above, the ethical component, which is based on the refusal of any food of animal origin, plays a lot in veganism. While for the plant based is not a purely moral and moralistic discourse but on the real thought of being able to keep healthy with the food discipline and be respectful of the environment surrounding us.

Plant based diet full shopping list. What to eat and what to avoid

Now we can examine the complete shopping list of the plant based diet.

Let's briefly summarize the principles on which this particular type of diet is based:

- Emphasizes whole, minimally processed foods.

- Limits or avoids animal products.

- Focuses on plants, including vegetables, fruits, whole grains, legumes, seeds and nuts, which should make up most of what you eat.

- Excludes refined foods, like added sugars, white flour and processed oils.

- Pays special attention to food quality, promoting locally sourced, organic food whenever possible.

As for what you can usually eat, we can say the general consumption of:

- Wholegrain and flours

- extra virgin olive oil

- Seasonal fruit and vegetables: these foods are the basis of every meal.

- In this diet you can also eat sweets but only and exclusively homemade and with controlled raw materials, simple and not very refined, preferably of vegetable origin - for example by replacing milk with soy or rice drinks, and eggs with other natural thickeners such as flaxseed, or simple ripe banana.

- You can also consume nuts and seeds.

As for absolutely forbidden foods, there are all those ready-made and processed:

- ready-made sauces
- chips
- biscuits
- various kinds of snacks
- sugary cereals,
- Spreads, snacks and many other notoriously unhealthy foods.
- Junk food and fast food are therefore absolutely banned
- Sugar beverages

Regarding the complete shopping list:

- Fruits: Berries, citrus fruits, pears, peaches, pineapple, bananas, etc.

- Vegetables: Kale, spinach, tomatoes, broccoli, cauliflower, carrots, asparagus, peppers, etc.

- Starchy vegetables: Potatoes, sweet potatoes, butternut squash, etc.

- Whole grains: Brown rice, rolled oats, spelt, quinoa, brown rice pasta, barley, etc.

- Healthy fats with omega 3: Avocados, olive oil, coconut oil, unsweetened coconut, etc.

- Legumes: Peas, chickpeas, lentils, peanuts, beans, black beans, etc.

- Seeds, nuts and nut butter: Almonds, cashews, macadamia nuts, pumpkin seeds, sunflower seeds, natural peanut butter, tahini, etc.

- Unsweetened plant-based milk: Coconut milk, almond milk, cashew milk, etc.

- Spices, herbs and seasonings: Basil, rosemary, turmeric, curry, black pepper, salt, etc.

- Condiments: Salsa, mustard, nutritional yeast, soy sauce, vinegar, lemon juice, etc.

- Plant-based protein: Tofu, tempeh, seitan, and plant based protein sources or powders with no added sugar or artificial ingredients.
- Beverages: Coffee, tea, sparkling water, etc.

There is the chance to add food of animal origin very rarely, for example if you have specific nutritional needs or if it has been strongly recommended by your doctor. Anyway, if supplementing your plant-based diet with animal products choose quality products from grocery stores or, better yet, purchase them from local farms.

- Eggs: Pasture-raised when possible.
- Poultry: Free-range, organic when possible.
- Beef and pork: Pastured or grass-fed when possible.
- Seafood: Wild-caught from sustainable fisheries when possible.
- Dairy: Organic dairy products from pasture-raised animals whenever possible.

Avocado and lime hummus

PREPARATION TIME: 5 minutes
REST TIME: 30 minutes in the fridge
COOKING TIME: 5 minutes
CALORIES: 260

INGREDIENTS FOR 4 SERVINGS

- 230 grams of drained chickpeas

- 2 ripe avocados

- 30 ml of extra virgin olive oil

- 25 grams of red onion

- 1 small lime

- 1 tablespoon of coriander powder or fresh parsley

- Salt to taste

DIRECTIONS

1. First, peel the avocados raw after removing the central woody stone.

2. Peel and slice the onion and peel the lime in order to keep only the pulp.

3. Pour all the ingredients, then add the boiled chickpeas, salt, oil and coriander, into a powerful blender and operate: you will need to obtain a cream with a smooth and homogeneous consistency.

4. Correct with salt if needed.

5. To have a coarser consistency, you can also blend only part of the avocado and mash the rest with the tines of a fork. Only then can you mix it with the rest of the cream.

6. Use the hummus to accompany your appetizers or simply serve alone.

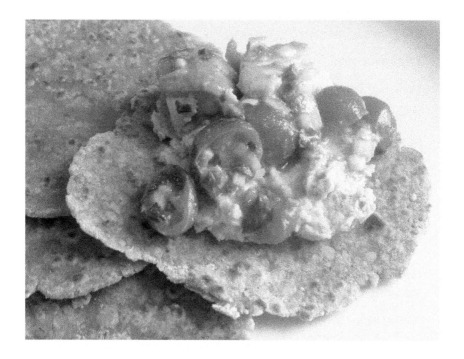

Spicy avocado orange hummus

PREPARATION TIME: 5 minutes
REST TIME: 30 minutes in the fridge
COOKING TIME: 5 minutes

CALORIES: 260

INGREDIENTS FOR 4 SERVINGS

- 230 grams of drained chickpeas

- 2 ripe avocados

- 1 pinch of chilli powder

- 30 ml of extra virgin olive oil

- 25 grams of shallot

- 1 orange

- 1 tablespoon of coriander powder or fresh parsley

- Salt to taste

DIRECTIONS

1. First, peel the avocados raw after removing the central woody stone.

2. Season avocado with chilli powder.

3. Peel and slice the shallot and peel the orange too in order to keep only the pulp.

4. Pour all the ingredients, then add the boiled chickpeas, salt, oil and coriander, into a powerful blender and operate: you will need to obtain a cream with a smooth and homogeneous consistency.

5. Correct with salt if needed.

6. To have a coarser consistency, you can also blend only part of the avocado and mash the rest with the tines of a fork. Only then can you mix it with the rest of the cream.

7. Use the hummus to accompany your appetizers or simply serve alone.

Fried bread with red lentils and mango humus

PREPARATION TIME: 5 minutes
COOKING TIME: 20 minutes
CALORIES: 490

INGREDIENTS FOR 4 SERVINGS

- 8 slices of soft wholemeal bread
- 200 grams of lentil and mango hummus cream (see recipe above)
- 180 grams of chickpeas flour
- 350 ml of water
- A few black cabbage leaves
- Wholemeal Bread crumbs homemade to taste
- Seeds oil

DIRECTIONS

1. Wash the black cabbage leaves well and remove the hard central rib.
2. After that sauté them for 5 minutes in a pan with a drop of oil and a pinch of salt to make them flavour.
3. Stuff 3 slices of bread with the hummus of red lentils and mango, cover with 2-3 black cabbage leaves and close the sandwiches with the other 3 slices of bread.
4. In a dish, pour the chickpea flour with water and a pinch of salt and mix well until the batter is smooth and without lumps.
5. In a second dish pour the breadcrumbs, then proceed to bread your sandwiches by passing them first in the batter and then in the

breadcrumbs, making sure to coat them in an even layer, especially along the edges.

6. Heat up the oil, and when it is hot, fry the sandwiches until golden and crunchy.

7. Drain them with a slotted spoon on a plate covered with paper towel so that they lose excess oil, then cut them in half, making two triangles from each and serve immediately hot.

Raisins coleslaw

PREPARATION TIME: 5 minutes
COOKING TIME: 5 minutes

CALORIES: 176

INGREDIENTS FOR 4 SERVINGS

- 2 carrots (180 grams about)
- 250 grams of cabbage
- ½ red apple
- 70 grams of raisins
- 90 grams of soy yogurt
- 90 grams of plant based mayonnaise (see basic recipe)
- 3 tablespoons of apple cider vinegar
- Salt and pepper to taste

DIRECTIONS

1. Soak the raisins first in hot water for 10-15 minutes, then drain and squeeze them to remove as much water as possible.
2. Meanwhile, peel the carrots, and then cut them into thin sticks.
3. Wash the apple well and cut it into slices first, then into sticks too, and finally thinly slice the cabbage as well.
4. Combine the vegetables and fruit in a bowl and season with the dressing prepared by mixing the soy yogurt, mayonnaise, apple cider vinegar, salt and pepper in a small bowl.
5. You can serve your raisins coleslaw immediately.

Cannellini beans and olive slices

PREPARATION TIME: 10 minutes
COOKING TIME: 20 minutes
CALORIES: 129

INGREDIENTS FOR 8 SERVINGS
- 250 grams of cooked cannellini beans
- 90 grams of corn starch
- 1 tablespoon of mustard
- 50 grams of green olives
- 1 tablespoon of tamari (gluten-free soy sauce)
- Salt and oil
- Homemade vegetable broth (see basic recipe)

DIRECTIONS
1. Rinse and dry the cannellini beans well, then transfer them to the food processor together with the olives, mustard, corn starch, tamari, a pinch of salt and a drizzle of extra virgin olive oil.
2. Blend everything well until you get a homogeneous mixture then transfer it to the refrigerator for at least 3 hours to make it firm up a little.
3. Transfer the dough to a clean white cloth, form a cylinder with the help of wet hands, roll it up in the cloth and tie the ends and the centre with kitchen twine.
4. Then immerse the cylinder in a large pot full of lightly salted boiling broth and cook for 20 minutes.

5. Once cooked, remove it from the broth and let it cool completely before serving cut into slices.

Quinoa pods

PREPARATION TIME: 15 minutes
COOKING TIME: 20 minutes
CALORIES: 112

INGREDIENTS FOR 4 SERVINGS

- 120 grams of quinoa
- 2 sheets of chopped nori seaweed
- Olive oil to taste
- Salt and Pepper To Taste

DIRECTIONS

1. Bring 400 ml of water to a boil.
2. Rinse the quinoa and let it drain.
3. Put the quinoa in the pot with boiling water, add the salt and cook for 15 minutes.
4. Now drain it and let it cool in a bowl.
5. Take a baking sheet and line it with parchment paper.
6. Now add salt, pepper, olive oil and the nori seaweed to the quinoa and mix.
7. Put the quinoa, with the help of a spoon, in the pan.
8. Press with the spoon until you have a thin enough layer.
9. Put in the oven and cook at 180 ° C for 10 minutes.
10. Remove the quinoa from the oven, let it rest for a couple of minutes, then cut it into squares and serve.

Spicy cauliflower

PREPARATION TIME: 5 minutes
COOKING TIME: 10 minutes

CALORIES: 65

INGREDIENTS FOR 4 SERVINGS

- 500 grams of cauliflower flowers

- 30 ml of olive oil

- 1 pinch of turmeric powder

- 1 pinch of garlic powder

- 2 grams of powder

- 1 pinch of powder

- Salt and black pepper to taste

DIRECTIONS

1. First, preheat the oven at 180 °C.

2. Meanwhile, clean the cauliflower and get only the flowers.

3. Put the cauliflower flowers in a bowl and drizzle with olive oil until all the cauliflower is well coated.

4. Mix the cauliflower with all the spices.

5. Add the cauliflower to a baking pan.

6. Cook it for about 10 minutes.

7. Serve the spiced cauliflower as soon as it has cooled.

Sweet potato and chicory toast

PREPARATION TIME: 5 minutes
COOKING TIME: 8minutes

CALORIES: 245

INGREDIENTS FOR 4 SERVINGS

- 1 large sweet potato
- ½ apple
- 2 tablespoons of almond cream (see basic recipe)
- 2 tablespoons of dried red fruits
- 3 tablespoons of chickpea hummus (see basic recipe)
- 100 grams of blanched chicory
- ½ lemon
- 1pinch of Chilli

DIRECTIONS

1. Rinse and peel the sweet potatoes.
2. With a very sharp knife cut them into slices about 4-5 mm thick, trying to get at least eight.
3. Put them in the toaster on maximum power for 5 minutes or until they are golden on the outside and soft on the inside.
4. Season the boiled chicory with salt, oil, a drop of lemon juice and a pinch of chilli.
5. Stuff half the sweet potato slices with a little chickpea hummus and the chicory for the savory version.

6. For the sweet version, on the other hand, spread each toast with a veil of almond cream and decorate with thin apple slices and red fruits.

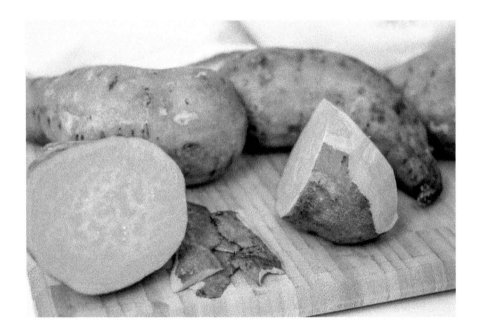

Edamame cream toast

PREPARATION TIME: 10 minutes
COOKING TIME: 5 minutes
CALORIES: 315

INGREDIENTS FOR 4 SERVINGS

- 8 slices of wholemeal bread
- 180 grams of edamame already cleaned
- 50 grams of rocket
- 50 grams of extra virgin olive oil
- 1 teaspoon of nutritional yeast
- ½ lemon
- 1 garlic clove

DIRECTIONS

1. First, peel the garlic clove.
2. Fry the garlic clove in a pan with a drop of oil and once it is golden add the edamame together with a pinch of salt and pepper, then leave them to cook over medium-low heat for 5-7 minutes with a lid until they will have softened.
3. Then turn off the flame and let them cool.
4. Transfer the edamame to the food processor and blend them coarsely, then transfer half of the edamame to a bowl and blend the remaining half with half of the rocket, extra virgin olive oil, nutritional yeast,

lemon zest and a tablespoon of lemon juice, until a homogeneous cream is obtained.

5. Coarsely chop the remaining rocket on a cutting board using a knife, and then add it to the edamame in the bowl together with the pureed cream.

6. Mix well to mix all the ingredients, and then serve the dip on slices of toasted bread.

Veggies Strudel

PREPARATION TIME: 30 minutes
COOKING TIME: 30/35 minutes

CALORIES: 310

INGREDIENTS FOR 4 SERVINGS

- 2 rolls of plant based puff pastry (see basic recipe)
- 1 carrot
- 3 zucchini
- 50 grams of fresh peas
- 15 grams of corn
- 120 grams of grated tofu cheese
- 40 ml of soymilk cream
- Soy butter
- Olive oil
- Salt and pepper

DIRECTIONS

1. Start with the vegetables.
2. Peel the carrot, wash it and then cut it into cubes.
3. Peel the zucchini, peel them, wash them and then cut them into cubes.
4. Wash fresh peas under running water and let them dry.
5. Take a pan and heat a drizzle of olive oil.
6. As soon as it is hot, put carrots, zucchini, peas and corn to brown.
7. Cook for 5 minutes, season with salt and pepper and then turn off.

8. Add the tofu cheese and soymilk cream to the vegetables and mix-to-mix everything.
9. Roll out the bread dough with a rolling pin trying to give it the shape of a rectangle.
10. Spread the vegetable filling inside and add a few knobs of butter spread over the filling.
11. Now roll the dough on itself.
12. Take a baking tray and brush it with a little oil.
13. Place the veggies strudel inside the baking pan.
14. Place the baking pan in the oven at 200ºC and let cook for 30 minutes about.
15. Check the cooking and, if cooked, take it out of the oven, otherwise continue for another 5/8 minutes.
16. As soon as it is cooked, take the strudel out of the oven, cut it into slices and serve immediately.

Zucchini and ricotta Strudel

PREPARATION TIME: 30 minutes

COOKING TIME: 30/35 minutes
CALORIES: 285

INGREDIENTS FOR 4 SERVINGS
1. 2 rolls of plant based puff pastry (see basic recipe)

2. 4 zucchini

3. 50 grams of green beans

4. 1 tbsp of corn

5. 120 grams of homemade ricotta cheese

6. 40 ml of soymilk cream

7. Soy butter

8. Olive oil

9. Salt and pepper

DIRECTIONS
1. Start with the vegetables.

2. Peel the zucchini, peel them, wash them and then cut them into cubes.

3. Wash green beans under running water and let them dry.

4. When they are dry, cut into little pieces.

5. Take a pan and heat a drizzle of olive oil.

6. As soon as it is hot, put zucchini green beans, and corn to brown.

7. Cook for 5 minutes, season with salt and pepper and then turn off.

8. Add the tofu cheese and soymilk cream to the vegetables and mix-to-mix everything.
9. Roll out the bread dough with a rolling pin trying to give it the shape of a rectangle.
10. Spread the vegetable filling inside and add a few knobs of butter spread over the filling.
11. Now roll the dough on itself.
12. Take a baking tray and brush it with a little oil.
13. Place the veggies strudel inside the baking pan.
14. Place the baking pan in the oven at 200ºC and let cook for 30 minutes about.
15. Check the cooking and, if cooked, take it out of the oven, otherwise continue for another 5/8 minutes.
16. As soon as it is cooked, take the strudel out of the oven, cut it into slices and serve immediately.

Zucchini and soy yogurt pie

PREPARATION TIME: 30 minutes
COOKING TIME: 30/35 minutes

CALORIES: 310

INGREDIENTS FOR 4 SERVINGS
- 1 roll of homemade shortcrust (patè briseè) pastry
- 1 jar of 200 grams of soy yogurt
- 2 zucchini
- 1 spring onion (green leaves only)
- Olive oil to taste
- Salt and pepper to taste

DIRECTIONS
1. Roll out the shortcrust pastry with parchment paper in a round pan.
2. Season the yogurt with oil, salt and pepper, and pour it over the shortcrust pastry levelling.
3. Coarsely chop the spring onion leaves, slice the zucchini, and arrange everything on top of the yogurt.
4. Season to taste with a drizzle of oil, a pinch of salt and pepper.
5. Fold the edges and bake at 180ºC for about 25 minutes (until the dough is golden brown).
6. Leave to cool for 5-10 minutes before cutting to allow the yogurt to set.
7. Serve still hot.

Tofu and zucchini plum cake

PREPARATION TIME: 30 minutes

COOKING TIME: 35 minutes
CALORIES: 310

INGREDIENTS FOR 4 SERVINGS
- 150 grams of wholemeal flour
- 25 grams of corn starch
- 120 ml of natural soy yogurt
- 130 ml of soymilk
- 80 ml of extra virgin olive oil
- 1 sachet of cream of tartar
- 2 large zucchini
- 1 stick of tofu
- 4–5 dried tomatoes
- basil and parsley to taste
- 3 tablespoons of low salt soy sauce

DIRECTIONS
1. First wash the zucchini well, and then remove the apex and the final part.
2. Before cutting them into cubes or washers, with the help of a potato peeler, create strips of peel that you will use to decorate the plum cake.
3. Take the tomatoes in oil, drain and cut them into small pieces.

4. Do the same with the tofu after blanching it in unsalted water to eliminate the bitter aftertaste that distinguishes it.

5. Put the zucchini in a pan with a drizzle of oil and a pinch of salt, halfway through cooking add the tomatoes, diced tofu and then, lastly, chopped parsley and basil.

6. Leave the "filling" aside. If the tofu is very wet or leaking water (depending on the brand) make sure to dry, the cubes with a little paper towel.

7. Meanwhile, prepare the dough.

8. In a large bowl put the flour, baking powder and corn starch, sifting everything.

9. Now add the liquids, then the soy yogurt, milk, oil and a couple of pinches of salt.

10. Start mixing until the mixture is soft and not lumpy, finally add the soy sauce and mix everything again.

11. Now add the previously prepared vegetable and tofu filling to the mixture and mix carefully trying to leave the ingredients intact.

12. Take the loaf pan and grease it lightly with a little oil or line it with parchment paper. Now decorate the surface of the plum cake with the strips of zucchini peel: you can decide to make small circles, curls, or lines, the important thing is that you put them sideways and let them sink halfway into the dough to make them stay still. Then bake everything at 200 ° for about 30/35 minutes in a static oven until the surface of the plum cake is golden brown. Inside, the plum cake will be very soft due to the presence of the zucchini and tofu.

13. You can serve it when it has cooled slightly.

Peas and asparagus plum cake

PREPARATION TIME: 10 minutes
COOKING TIME: 55 minutes

CALORIES: 206

INGREDIENTS FOR 4 SERVINGS

- 500 grams of asparagus
- 500 grams of fresh peas
- 2 fresh spring onions
- 200 grams of chickpea flour
- 300 ml of water
- A handful of pumpkin seeds
- 3 tablespoons of olive oil
- Curry to taste
- Salt and pepper to taste

DIRECTIONS

1. Clean and boil the asparagus in water for 15 minutes.

2. In a separate pot, boil the peas in water (15 minutes from when the water starts to boil). Use 300 ml of the asparagus cooking water and mix it with the chickpea flour, then add the oil, salt, pepper and curry.

3. Once everything is well blended with a whisk, add the cut asparagus (in 3 or 4 pieces, depending on their size), chopped spring onions and peas.

4. Take a loaf pan, line it with baking paper (previously wet and wrung out), pour the mixture into it and cook it on the last shelf in a preheated oven at 200 ° C for 30-40 minutes.

5. Serve still hot.

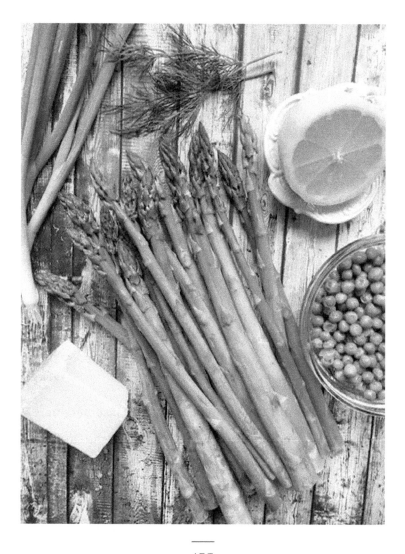

Almond cheese asparagus

PREPARATION TIME: 20 minutes
COOKING TIME: 20 minutes
CALORIES: 200

INGREDIENTS FOR 4 SERVINGS

- 1 pound asparagus

- 10 ml of olive oil

- 1 tablespoon minced onions

- 3 tablespoon chopped thyme

- 100 ml of soymilk cream

- 100 grams of creamy almond cheese

- 2 teaspoon of warm water

- 1 cup of soy butter

DIRECTIONS

1. Wash and chop onions.

2. Combine the oil, onions, in the saucepan and bring to a boil over medium-high heat.

3. Cook until reduced by two thirds (about 3 minutes).

4. Remove the saucepan from the heat and strain the sauce into a heatproof bowl.

5. Add the soymilk cream and water and whisk to incorporate.

6. Set the bowl over a pan with simmering water on the stovetop and continue to whisk until the egg starts to thicken (2–3 minutes).

7. Remove the bowl from the heat and slowly drizzle a little of the soy butter into the bowl while whisking constantly to incorporate.

8. Continue this on the heat, off-the-heat pattern until all the soy butter is incorporated.

9. Season with the salt and pepper, and add the almond cheese.

10. Keep the sauce warm while you cook the asparagus (do not allow the sauce to boil or it will separate).

11. Place the asparagus in the baking pan. Pour over the sauce

12. Place in the oven at 190° C.

13. Cook for about 15/20 minutes.

14. When the cooking time is complete, transfer the asparagus to a serving plate, and serve still hot.

Tofu and figs canapés

PREPARATION TIME: 15 minutes

COOKING TIME: 5 minutes
CALORIES: 360

INGREDIENTS FOR 3 SERVINGS

- 6 slices of whole wheat bread
- 120 grams of tofu
- 65 ml of unsweetened soymilk
- 5 grams of capers
- 1 handful of rocket
- 4–5 figs
- 2 sprigs of fresh thyme
- 1 pinch of garlic powder
- Salt and pepper to taste
- 1 tbsp olive oil

DIRECTIONS

1. First, prepare rocket tofu cream.
2. Wash the rocket and let it dry.
3. Cut tofu into pieces.
4. Now, blend the tofu, soymilk, capers, garlic powder, salt, pepper and a dash of oil in a food processor until smooth.

5. Finally, add the rocket and operate the chopper again just a few seconds to incorporate the rocket into the cream, but without chopping it.
6. Then, prepare the canapés.
7. Wash the figs well and cut them into slices about 4-5 mm thick and set aside.
8. Lightly grease each slice of bread and fill it with a nice layer of rocket cream, a few slices of figs and a few leaves of fresh thyme.
9. Arrange your canapés on a baking pan and bake in a static oven at 200° C for 5 minutes.
10. Remove from the oven, allow to cool slightly and serve

Eggplant and herbs cream canapés

PREPARATION TIME: 20 minutes

COOKING TIME: 10 minutes
CALORIES: 320

INGREDIENTS FOR 6 SERVINGS
- 12 slices of whole wheat bread
- 1 eggplant
- 1 garlic clove
- ½ teaspoon of dried mixed herbs
- ½ teaspoon of paprika
- 1 handful of fresh rocket
- 2 tablespoons of sesame seeds
- extra virgin olive oil

DIRECTIONS
1. First, peel the eggplants (we remove the peel to make the cream completely smooth and homogeneous).
2. Cut them into cubes and sauté them in a pan with the clove of garlic, a drop of oil, the mixed herbs, paprika and salt. Leave them first cook with the lid on for a few minutes and then remove it, proceeding over medium heat until the pulp of the eggplants is very soft.
3. Now you just have to blend the cooked eggplants until you get a smooth and homogeneous cream.

4. Spread the cream on the bread (if you want, you can also heat it a little in a pan to make it crunchy) and decorate with fresh rocket leaves and sesame seeds.

5. You can serve your canapés.

Basil and tofu cream canapés

PREPARATION TIME: 20 minutes

COOKING TIME: 10 minutes
CALORIES: 320

INGREDIENTS FOR 6 SERVINGS

- 12 slices of whole wheat bread
- 150 grams of tofu cheese in a stick
- 1 handful of fresh basil
- 1 organic lemon (juice and zest)
- 2 tablespoons of walnuts
- salt and pepper to taste
- olive oil to taste

DIRECTIONS

1. Start by washing basil leaves.
2. Let them dry.
3. Cube tofu cheese and put all ingredients in a mixer.
4. Blend the tofu after adding the well washed and dried leaves of fresh basil, the juice and the lemon zest to the mixer.
5. Also, add salt and pepper to the cream: you will have to obtain, even in this case, a homogeneous mixture.
6. Spread your canapés with the cream, decorate with lemon zest, and roughly chopped walnut kernels.

Artichokes and tofu cream canapés

PREPARATION TIME: 20 minutes

COOKING TIME: 10 minutes
CALORIES: 345

INGREDIENTS FOR 6 SERVINGS
- 12 slices of whole wheat bread
- 140 grams of artichokes in oil
- 90 grams of classic tofu in a stick
- 1 pinch of garlic powder
- ½ teaspoon of dried mint or 4/5 fresh mint leaves
- 1 teaspoon of apple cider vinegar
- 150 grams of mixed herbs
- 2 tablespoons of cashews

DIRECTIONS
1. Take the artichokes in oil and drain them very well, in order to eliminate the excess oil. You can choose the type of artichoke you prefer.
2. Now, cut the tofu stick into cubes and put it in the mixer.
3. Then add a pinch of powdered or dried garlic (less indigestible, but with a strong flavour), the dried mint (if you use fresh eye to the quantities, it is quite strong), artichokes and vinegar: blend everything until you get a cream with a homogeneous consistency and add salt if necessary.
4. Now let us prepare the decoration of the canapés.
5. Separately, sauté the fresh or frozen herbs in a pan with a little salt, oil and a pinch of garlic: let them dry without flaking.

6. Then chop the cashews with a knife coarsely.

7. Spread the artichoke cream on the slices of bread, place the sautéed herbs on top and sprinkle with cashews.

Tofu and avocado canapés

PREPARATION TIME: 15 minutes

COOKING TIME: 5 minutes
CALORIES: 360

INGREDIENTS FOR 3 SERVINGS
- 6 slices of whole wheat bread
- 120 grams of tofu
- 65 ml of unsweetened almond milk
- 5 grams of capers
- 1 handful of lettuce
- Half of avocado
- 2 sprigs of fresh thyme
- 1 pinch of garlic powder
- Salt and pepper to taste
- 1 tbsp olive oil

DIRECTIONS
1. First, prepare lettuce tofu cream.
2. Wash the rocket and let it dry.
3. Cut tofu into pieces.
4. Now, blend the tofu, lettuce, almond milk, capers, garlic powder, salt, pepper and a dash of oil in a food processor until smooth.
5. Meanwhile peel and wash half avocado, removing the core and slice it.
6. Make slices of about 4-5 mm thick and set aside.
7. Then, prepare the canapés

8. Lightly grease each slice of bread and fill it with a nice layer of lettuce tofu cream, a few slices of avocado and a few leaves of fresh thyme.

9. Arrange your canapés on a baking pan and bake in a static oven at 200° C for 5 minutes.

10. Remove from the oven, allow to cool slightly and serve

Soy cheese and cucumber canapés

PREPARATION TIME: 15 minutes
COOKING TIME: 5 minutes

CALORIES: 360

INGREDIENTS FOR 3 SERVINGS

- 6 slices of whole wheat bread
- 120 grams of soy cheese
- 65 ml of unsweetened soymilk
- 1 handful of rocket
- 1 pinch of nutmeg
- 1 cucumber
- 2 sprigs of fresh thyme
- 1 pinch of garlic powder
- Salt and pepper to taste
- 1 tbsp olive oil

DIRECTIONS

1. First, prepare rocket cheese cream.
2. Wash the rocket and let it dry.
3. Cut tofu into pieces.
4. Now, blend the soy cheese, soymilk, nutmeg, garlic powder, salt, pepper and a dash of oil in a food processor until smooth.

5. Finally, add the rocket and operate the chopper again just a few seconds to incorporate the rocket into the cream, but without chopping it.
6. Then, prepare the canapés.
7. Wash the cucumber, peel and cut it into slices about 4-5 mm thick and set aside.
8. Lightly grease each slice of bread and fill it with a nice layer of rocket cream, a few slices of cucumber and a few leaves of fresh thyme.
9. Arrange your canapés on a baking pan and bake in a static oven at 200° C for 5 minutes.
10. Remove from the oven, allow to cool slightly and serve

Avocado and rice milk cream

PREPARATION TIME: 10 minutes

CALORIES: 130

INGREDIENTS FOR 4 SERVINGS

- 1 avocado
- sesame oil to taste
- 100 ml of rice milk
- juice of one lime to taste
- Salt to taste.
- extra virgin olive oil to taste
- chili pepper to taste

DIRECTIONS

1. To make the avocado and rice milk cream, choose a ripe avocado with a firm, green flesh.
2. Cut your avocado in half and remove the stone. Then, remove the pulp, using a teaspoon and cut it into cubes.
3. Squeeze the lime to obtain the juice and pour it together with the avocado into the glass of the hand blender.
4. Add the extra virgin olive oil, a pinch of salt and the rice milk.
5. Blend for a long time to obtain a perfectly smooth sauce.
6. Then add the chilli, adjusting the degree of spiciness to your taste, mix well. You can directly serve your avocado and rice milk cream.

Spiced soy avocado

PREPARATION TIME: 15 minutes

COOKING TIME: 15 minutes
CALORIES: 350

INGREDIENTS FOR 4 SERVINGS

- 4 avocados cut into thick wedges
- 40 grams of wholemeal breadcrumbs
- 2 grams of garlic powder
- 2 grams of onions powder
- 10 grams of smoked paprika
- 1 gram of cayenne pepper
- Salt and pepper to taste.
- 60 grams of wholemeal flour
- 100 ml of soymilk cream
- saffron mayonnaise (see basic recipe)

DIRECTIONS

1. Cut the avocados into wedges about 25mm thick.
2. Combine the breadcrumbs, garlic powder, onion powder, smoked paprika, cayenne pepper, salt and pepper in a bowl.
3. Dig each wedge of avocado into the flour, then dip it in the soymilk cream and roll it into the breadcrumb mixture.
4. Preheat the oven 200° C.
5. Put the avocados in a baking pan.

6. Grease the baking pan a little oil before adding the avocados.

7. Cook at 200° C for about 15 minutes

8. Flip the avocados halfway through cooking.

9. Serve warm with saffron mayonnaise.

Avocado chips with paprika mayonnaise

PREPARATION TIME: 10 minutes

COOKING TIME: 20 minutes
CALORIES: 272

INGREDIENTS FOR 4 SERVINGS
- 1 avocado
- 50 grams of rice flour
- 70 ml water
- 50 grams of wholemeal breadcrumbs
- Salt and pepper to taste
- Paprika mayonnaise for serving

DIRECTIONS
1. Cut in half the avocado.
2. Remove the central stone and with the help of a spoon remove the peel.
3. Cut the avocado into slices that are not too thin. In a bowl, dissolve the rice flour with the water, mixing well with a whisk to remove all possible lumps.
4. Season with salt and pepper. In a second bowl, pour the breadcrumbs instead.
5. Pass the avocado slices first in the rice flour batter, then in the breadcrumbs and arrange them on a baking sheet lined with parchment paper.

6. Once all the avocado slices have been breaded, bake them in a static oven at 180 ° C for 20 minutes, seasoning them first with a drop of oil to make them golden.
7. Once ready, serve hot or at most lukewarm, accompanied by paprika mayonnaise

Pasta and cereals

Wholemeal penne with seitan and hazelnuts

PREPARATION TIME: 10 minutes
COOKING TIME: 20 minutes

CALORIES: 353

INGREDIENTS FOR 4 SERVINGS

- 320 grams of wholemeal penne pasta
- 100 grams of seitan
- 1 onion
- 1 red bell pepper
- 1 yellow bell pepper
- 1 tablespoon of soy sauce
- Olive oil to taste
- Salt and pepper to taste

DIRECTIONS

1. Start by putting water and salt in a saucepan and bring to a boil.
2. Cut the peppers in half and remove the white filaments and seeds. Wash them and cut them into cubes.
3. Peel the onion and wash it. Then chop it.

4. Dab the seitan with absorbent paper and then cut it into cubes.

5. Put a tablespoon of oil in a pan to heat. When hot, put the onion to brown for a couple of minutes.

6. Add the peppers and let them sauté for 3 minutes.

7. Add the seitan and cook for another minute. Stir, season with salt and pepper and turn off.

8. When the water starts to boil, cook the pasta.

9. Cook for 10 minutes and then drain.

10. Put it in the pan with the sauce, stir to flavour well, then put it on plates and serve.

Wholemeal spaghetti in red bell pepper sauce

PREPARATION TIME: 10 minutes

COOKING TIME: 20 minutes
CALORIES: 380

INGREDIENTS FOR 4 SERVINGS
- 320 grams of wholemeal spaghetti
- 3 bell red peppers
- 1shallot
- 1 garlic cloves
- 120 ml of soy cream milk
- Olive oil to taste
- Salt and pepper to taste

DIRECTIONS
1. Divide the bell peppers in half, wash them, and remove the seeds and white filaments.
2. Heat a grill and put the peppers to grill for 4 minutes per side.
3. Put the peppers in a bowl and let them cool.
4. Meanwhile, put a saucepan with water and salt to boil.
5. Peel and wash the garlic and shallots and then chop them.
6. As soon as the peppers are cold, peel them and cut them into slices.
7. Heat a tablespoon of oil in a pan and sauté the garlic and shallots.
8. After two minutes, add the peppers and cream.
9. Cook for 2 minutes, stirring constantly.
10. Season with salt and pepper and turn off.

11. When the water starts to boil, put the pasta to cook for 10 minutes.

12. Now drain the pasta and put it in the pan with the peppers.

13. Stir, let flavour well and then put on plates.

14. You can serve.

Vegetarian dim sum

PREPARATION TIME: 15 minutes
COOKING TIME: 40 minutes

CALORIES: 304

INGREDIENTS FOR 4 SERVINGS

- 500 grams of rice flour
- 300 ml of water
- 2 red peppers
- 1 large carrot
- 3 shallots
- 2 medium zucchini
- 1 chilli
- 100 ml of soy sauce
- Salt and Pepper To Taste.
- Olive oil to taste
- 15 strands of chives

DIRECTIONS

1. Start with the dough. In a planetary mixer put the flour and a pinch of salt.
2. Operate the planetary mixer at minimum speed and start pouring the water flush.
3. Knead for about 10 minutes, until, in practice, you get a smooth and elastic mixture.

4. Form the dough into a ball; wrap it in cling film and leave to rest for 60 minutes in the fridge.
5. Meanwhile, prepare the vegetables.
6. Remove the top cap from the peppers, cut them in half, remove the seeds and white filaments and then wash them. Cut them into very small cubes.
7. Peel and wash the carrot and shallots and then chop them.
8. Wash the zucchinis and then cut them into small cubes.
9. In a pan, heat a tablespoon of olive oil, and when it is hot enough, cook the vegetables.
10. Cook for about 8 minutes, long enough for them to soften.
11. Season with salt and pepper and turn off. Leave the vegetables to cool.
12. Now prepare the dim sum.
13. Take a piece of dough and roll it out with a rolling pin, helping yourself with a little flour, until you have a thin sheet (but not transparent otherwise when you go to close they will break).
14. With a pastry cutter or a glass, make a disc 8 cm in diameter.
15. Put a spoonful of vegetables in the centre and begin to pinch the edges bringing them towards the centre, forming folds. Continue until the pasta is used up.
16. Steam the Dim Sums for about 20 minutes.
17. Meanwhile, prepare the soy sauce.
18. Wash the chilli and then chop it.
19. Wash and chop the chives
20. Put the soy sauce in a bowl and add the chilli and chives.
21. Stir and set aside.

22. When the dim sum are cooked, put them immediately on the serving plates, sprinkle them with the soy sauce and serve.

Wholemeal macaroni with broccoli and basil

PREPARATION TIME: 20 minutes
COOKING TIME: 40 minutes

CALORIES: 545

INGREDIENTS FOR 4 SERVINGS

- 320 grams of wholemeal macaroni
- 600 grams of broccoli
- 10 basil leaves
- 1 plant based mozzarella
- 300 ml of plant based béchamel
- Salt and pepper to taste
- Olive oil to taste

DIRECTIONS

1. Remove the stem from the broccoli and keep only the flowers. Wash them and let them drain,
2. Boil a pot with plenty of water and salt.
3. As soon as it starts to boil, put the broccoli to cook.
4. Cook for 8 minutes, then drain and set aside.
5. In the same water as the broccoli, cook the pasta for another 8 minutes.
6. Drain it and keep the pasta aside.
7. Wash and dry the basil leaves.
8. Put the broccoli, pasta and béchamel in a bowl. Stir to flavour everything well.

9. Take a baking tray and brush it with olive oil.

10. Pour the pasta into the pan. Put the mozzarella cut into thin slices on top of the pasta.

11. Sprinkle with the basil leaves and then bake in the oven at 200 ° C for 15 minutes.

12. As soon as it is cooked, take it out of the oven, put it on serving plates and serve immediately.

Potato gnocchi with asparagus and peas

PREPARATION TIME: 20 minutes

COOKING TIME: 30 minutes
CALORIES: 405

INGREDIENTS FOR 4 SERVINGS

- 600 grams of homemade potato gnocchi
- 150 grams of asparagus
- 150 grams of peas
- 1 shallot
- Olive oil to taste
- Salt and pepper to taste

DIRECTIONS

1. Start by boiling plenty of water and salt.
2. Meanwhile, remove the stalk and the hardest part of the asparagus and then wash them.
3. Cut them in half lengthwise,
4. Peel and wash the shallot and then cut it into thin slices.
5. Rinse the peas and let them drain.
6. Heat a tablespoon of olive oil in a pan and as soon as it is hot, add the shallot.
7. Cook it for 2 minutes. Now put the peas. Stir sauté for 5 minutes and then add the asparagus and 40 ml of water.
8. Cook for 10 minutes, then season with salt and pepper and turn

off.

9. Now put the gnocchi to cook. The gnocchi will be cooked when they all rise to the surface.

10. Drain and put them in the pan with the vegetables.

11. Stir, cook well and then put them on plates and serve.

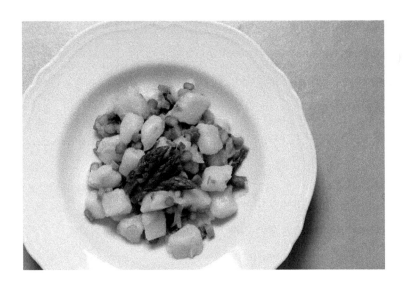

Pumpkin gnocchi with soy butter and sage

PREPARATION TIME: 10 minutes
COOKING TIME: 15 minutes

CALORIES: 350

INGREDIENTS FOR 4 SERVINGS

- 800 grams of homemade pumpkin gnocchi
- 50 grams of soy butter
- 6 sage leaves
- Salt and pepper to taste

DIRECTIONS

1. Take to boil a pot with plenty of water and salt.
2. As soon as it comes to a boil, put the pumpkin gnocchi to cook, a little at a time.
3. The gnocchi will be ready when they all rise to the surface.
4. As soon as they are ready, drain and set aside.
5. Wash and dry the sage leaves.
6. Put the butter in a non-stick pan and, when it has melted, put the sage leaves.
7. Cook for 3 minutes. Season with salt and pepper and then put the gnocchi in the pan.
8. Cook for a minute then turn off.
9. Put the gnocchi on serving plates and serve.

Wholemeal tagliatelle with bean cream

PREPARATION TIME: 10 minutes
COOKING TIME: 15 minutes
CALORIES: 520

INGREDIENTS FOR 4 SERVINGS

- 320 grams of wholemeal tagliatelle

- 400 grams of cooked beans

- 2 onions

- 4 tablespoons of tomato sauce

- 8 mint leaves

- Olive oil to taste

- Salt and pepper to taste

DIRECTIONS

1. Start by putting plenty of water and salt to boil.

2. Meanwhile, peel and wash the onions and then chop them.

3. Put two tablespoons of olive oil in a pan. When it is hot, brown the onion.

4. Cook it for 10 minutes, stirring often and then add the beans and tomato puree.

5. Season with salt and pepper, stir and continue cooking for another 5 minutes.

6. At this point, turn off, put all the contents of the pan in the glass of the blender and blend until you get a smooth and homogeneous cream.

7. Put the cream obtained in a bowl.

8. When the water has come to a boil, put the noodles to cook.

9. Cook for 10 minutes and then drain.

10. Put the noodles in the bowl with the bean cream and mix well to flavour everything.

11. Put the noodles on serving plates and serve.

Couscous with mushrooms and peas

PREPARATION TIME: 20 minutes
COOKING TIME: 25 minutes

CALORIES: 240

INGREDIENTS FOR 4 SERVINGS

- 300 grams of couscous
- 200 grams of peas
- 1 litre of vegetable broth
- 200 grams of mushrooms
- 1 clove of garlic
- 1 chilli
- 1 sprig of chopped parsley
- Olive oil to taste
- Salt and pepper to taste

DIRECTIONS

1. Remove the earthy part of the mushrooms, wash and dry them, then cut them into slices.
2. Peel and wash the garlic, then chop it.
3. Wash the peas and let them drain.
4. Put a tablespoon of olive oil in a pan and as soon as it is hot, brown the garlic.
5. When it is golden brown, add the mushrooms.
6. Stir, season with salt, pepper, and cook for 10 minutes.
7. Meanwhile, put the broth in a saucepan and bring to a boil. Now

put the peas to cook for 5 minutes, then drain them and keep them aside.

8. Put the couscous in another pan with a tablespoon of oil to toast for 3 minutes, stirring constantly to prevent it from burning.
9. Now add the peas, mushrooms, and mix.
10. Season with salt and pepper and then add 6 ladles of broth.
11. Lower the heat and cook until the broth is completely absorbed.
12. When the couscous is cooked, turn it off and put it on serving plates.
13. Season with a drizzle of oil, sprinkle with chopped parsley and serve.

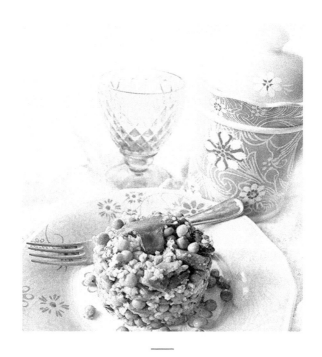

Zucchini noodles with baked tofu

PREPARATION TIME: 20 minutes
COOKING TIME: 10 minutes

CALORIES: 414

INGREDIENTS FOR 4 SERVINGS

- 4 zucchinis
- 300 grams of tofu
- 150 grams of cherry tomatoes
- 12 zucchini flowers
- 12 radishes
- 1 teaspoon of oregano
- 1 tablespoon of lemon juice
- 1 clove of garlic
- Salt and pepper to taste
- Olive oil to taste

DIRECTIONS

1. Wash the cherry tomatoes and then cut them into wedges.
2. Wash the zucchini flowers and then cut it into small pieces.
3. Wash the radishes and then cut them into slices.
4. Rinse the tofu and then pat it dry with absorbent paper.
5. Take a baking tray and brush it with olive oil.
6. Place the tofu in the centre of the pan and surround it with the cherry tomatoes and zucchini flowers.
7. Season everything with olive oil, oregano, salt and pepper.

8. Bake in the oven for 10 minutes at 180 ° C.

9. In the meantime, wash the zucchinis and with the special tool cut them into spaghetti.

10. Put them in a bowl and season with oil, salt and the juice of half a lemon.

11. As soon as the tofu is ready, take it out of the oven and place it together with the cherry tomatoes and zucchini flowers in a large serving dish.

12. Now put the zucchini spaghetti and put on the table.

Wholemeal pasta with seitan sauce

PREPARATION TIME: 20 minutes

COOKING TIME: 40 minutes
CALORIES: 440

INGREDIENTS FOR 4 SERVINGS

- 280 grams of wholemeal pasta
- 250 grams of tomato pulp
- 1 shallot
- 1 clove of garlic
- 1 tablespoon of soy sauce
- 200 grams of seitan
- 1 carrot
- 1 stick of celery
- The zest of one lemon
- 400 ml of vegetable broth
- 2 chopped sage leaves
- Salt and Pepper To Taste.
- Olive oil to taste

DIRECTIONS
1. Peel the garlic and onion and chop them.
2. Peel the carrot, wash it and chop it.
3. Remove the celery stalk and filaments, wash it and chop it.
4. Rinse and pat the seitan with absorbent paper and then chop it.

5. Put a tablespoon of olive oil in a saucepan and sauté garlic, shallot, celery and carrot.

6. Mix well and then add the sage.

7. After a couple of minutes, add the seitan.

8. Add the soy sauce, mix and let it absorb.

9. When it is absorbed, add the tomato pulp.

10. Season with salt and pepper and then add the vegetable broth.

11. Cook the ragù for 30 minutes.

12. Meanwhile, prepare the pasta.

13. Boil the water and salt and then cook the pasta following the cooking times shown in the package.

14. When it is ready, drain it and put it in the pot with the sauce.

15. Stir to flavour well, then put it on plates and serve.

Wholemeal penne with broccoli, cauliflower and almonds

PREPARATION TIME: 20 minutes

COOKING TIME: 30 minutes
CALORIES: 360

INGREDIENTS FOR 4 SERVINGS
- 320 grams of wholemeal penne
- 12 cauliflower flowers
- 12 broccoli flowers
- A clove of garlic
- A spoonful of sliced almonds
- Olive oil to taste
- Salt and Pepper to taste

DIRECTIONS
1. Wash the broccoli and cauliflower flowers. Steam them for about 15 minutes.
2. Meanwhile, put water and salt in a saucepan and bring to a boil. Now add the pasta and cook it following the instructions on the package.
3. Peel and wash the garlic and then cut it into thin slices.
4. Put a tablespoon of oil in a pan and when it is hot, put the garlic to brown.
5. Now add the almonds and sauté them for a minute then add the

vegetables.

6. Season with salt and pepper, cook them for a couple of minutes and then turn off.

7. Now drain the pasta and put it in the pan with the vegetables. Stir, season well then put the pasta on serving plates and serve.

Quinoa with tempeh and vegetables

PREPARATION TIME: 15 minutes + 20 minutes of marinating
COOKING TIME: 20 minutes
CALORIES: 237

INGREDIENTS FOR 4 SERVINGS

- 200 grams of cooked quinoa
- 160 grams of tempeh
- 8 cherry tomatoes
- 4 radishes
- 1 shallot
- 1 fennel
- 1 lemon
- 1 clove of garlic
- 3 teaspoons of honey
- 1 teaspoon of cumin seeds
- Olive oil to taste
- Salt and pepper to taste

DIRECTIONS

1. Dab the tempeh with absorbent paper and then cut it into slices.
2. Peel and wash the garlic and then chop it.
3. Wash and dry the lemon and grate the zest. Strain the juice into a bowl.
4. Put it in a bowl and season with cumin, minced garlic, salt, pepper,

honey, oil and grated lemon zest.

5. Leave to marinate for 20 minutes.

6. Now heat a plate and put the tempeh to grill for 3 minutes per side.

7. As soon as they are cooked, place the slices on a cutting board and cut them into strips.

8. Now wash the cherry tomatoes and cut them in half.

9. Wash the radishes and cut them into slices.

10. Peel the shallot, wash it and cut it into slices.

11. Wash the fennel and cut it into slices.

12. Put the quinoa in a bowl, add the vegetables and season everything with oil, salt, pepper and lemon juice.

13. Add the tempeh and mix to flavour everything well.

14. Now you can serve.

Quinoa with pumpkin, hazelnuts and coriander

PREPARATION TIME: 20 minutes
COOKING TIME: 15minutes
CALORIES: 215

INGREDIENTS FOR 4 SERVINGS

- 250 grams of quinoa
- 400 grams of pumpkin pulp
- 800 ml of vegetable broth
- 4 cloves of garlic
- 40 grams of hazelnuts
- 6 coriander leaves
- 2 teaspoons of cumin
- Salt and Pepper to taste
- Olive oil to taste

DIRECTIONS

1. Wash the pumpkin pulp and then cut it into small pieces.
2. Peel the garlic cloves and wash them.
3. Heat a tablespoon of oil in a saucepan and brown the garlic cloves.
4. Now add the quinoa and let it flavour for a couple of minutes.
5. At this point, pour half the broth and mix.
6. Add the pumpkin and cumin and continue mixing.
7. As soon as the broth is completely absorbed, add the rest.
8. Cook for another 15 minutes, stirring often.
9. Meanwhile, wash the coriander and chop it.

10. Also, chop the hazelnuts.

11. As soon as it is cooked, put the quinoa on the plates, sprinkle with the coriander and hazelnuts and serve.

Quinoa tomato and basil

PREPARATION TIME: 10 minutes+15 minutes to rest
COOKING TIME: 15minutes

CALORIES: 147

INGREDIENTS FOR 4 SERVINGS

- 300 grams of quinoa
- 16 cherry tomatoes
- 8 basil leaves
- Olive oil to taste
- Salt and Pepper to taste

DIRECTIONS

1. Rinse the quinoa under running water and then let it drain.
2. Bring 600 ml of water with salt to a boil and then cook the quinoa for 15 minutes.
3. After 15 minutes turn off, put the lid on the pot and let the quinoa rest for 15 minutes.
4. Meanwhile, wash the cherry tomatoes and cut them into 4 wedges.
5. Wash and dry the basil leaves.
6. Now put the quinoa in a bowl.
7. Add the cherry tomatoes and basil.
8. Season with salt, pepper and olive oil.
9. Mix well to flavour everything and serve.

Carrot gnocchi with mushroom sauce

PREPARATION TIME: 15 minutes
COOKING TIME: 20 minutes
CALORIES: 375

INGREDIENTS FOR 4 SERVINGS

- 600 grams of carrot gnocchi
- 350 grams of mixed mushrooms
- 1 clove of garlic
- 1 shallot
- 1 sprig of chopped parsley
- Salt and Pepper to taste.
- Olive oil to taste

DIRECTIONS

1. Put water and salt in a saucepan and bring to a boil.
2. Meanwhile, prepare the mushrooms.
3. Remove the earthy part of the mushrooms and then rinse them quickly under running water and dry them with a kitchen towel. Now cut them into thin slices.
4. Peel and wash the garlic and shallots and then chop them.
5. Heat two tablespoons of oil in a pan and as soon as it is hot, brown the garlic and shallots.
6. As soon as they are golden brown, add the parsley and mix.
7. Sauté for a minute and then add the mushrooms.
8. Stir, season with salt, pepper, and cook for 10 minutes. After the

cooking time, turn off and set aside.

9. When the water has come to a boil, add the gnocchi.

10. Cook them until they have all come to the surface, then drain and put them in the pan with the mushrooms.

11. Stir to flavour everything well. Put the gnocchi on serving plates and serve.

Carrot gnocchi with tomato sauce and capers

PREPARATION TIME: 20 minutes
COOKING TIME: 30 minutes

CALORIES: 299

INGREDIENTS FOR 4 SERVINGS

- 600 grams of homemade carrot dumplings

- 250 grams of organic tomato pulp

- 1 shallot

- 4 sage leaves

- A spoonful of capers

DIRECTIONS

1. Bring a saucepan with plenty of water and salt to a boil.

2. Meanwhile, prepare the tomato sauce. Wash and dry the sage leaves.

3. Peel and wash the shallot and then chop it.

4. Put a tablespoon of oil in a pan and when it is hot, put the shallot to fry for a couple of minutes.

5. Add the capers, sage, and mix well.

6. Sauté for a minute and then add the tomatoes. Season with salt and pepper, stir and cook for 12 minutes. As soon as ready, turn off and set aside.

7. When the water has boiled, put the carrot gnocchi inside.

8. Cook them until all the gnocchi have come to the surface.

9. Drain the gnocchi and put them in the pan with the sauce.

10. Stir to flavour well, put the gnocchi on serving plates and serve.

Potato gnocchi with asparagus cream

PREPARATION TIME: 20 minutes
COOKING TIME: 35 minutes
CALORIES: 259

INGREDIENTS FOR 4 SERVINGS

- 600 grams of potato gnocchi
- 300 ml of vegetable broth
- 1 onion
- 500 grams of asparagus
- Olive oil to taste
- Salt and Pepper to taste.

DIRECTIONS

1. Start by putting water and salt in a saucepan and bring to a boil.
2. Now switch to the asparagus.
3. Remove the stalk and the hardest parts of the asparagus and then wash them. Cut off the tips and set them aside. Cut the stem into small pieces.
4. Peel and wash the onion and then chop it.
5. Heat a tablespoon of oil in a saucepan. When it is hot, brown the onion.
6. Add the asparagus stalks and mix.
7. Cook for 5 minutes and then add the vegetable broth. Cook over low heat for 15 minutes. After 15 minutes, season with salt and pepper and turn off. Blend everything with an immersion blender.

8. In a pan, heat a tablespoon of oil and sauté the asparagus tips for 3 minutes.
9. When the water has come to a boil, pour the gnocchi and cook them until they all float to the surface.
10. Drain and put them in the pot with the asparagus cream. Stir until they are well incorporated.
11. Put the gnocchi on serving plates, sprinkle them with the asparagus tips and serve.

Potato gnocchi with mushrooms and cherry tomatoes

PREPARATION TIME: 20 minutes
COOKING TIME: 30 minutes
CALORIES: 259

INGREDIENTS FOR 4 SERVINGS

- 600 grams of homemade potato gnocchi
- 300 grams of mushrooms
- 2 tomatoes
- 1 clove of garlic
- A sprig of chopped parsley
- Olive oil to taste
- Salt and pepper to taste

DIRECTIONS

1. Boil a pot with water and salt.
2. Meanwhile, prepare the sauce. Remove the earthy part of the mushrooms, wash and dry them, then cut them into slices.
3. Peel and wash the garlic and then chop it.
4. Wash the tomatoes and then cut them into cubes.
5. Heat a tablespoon of oil in a pan and as soon as it is hot, brown the garlic.
6. Add the parsley and sauté for a minute, and then add the mushrooms.
7. Stir, season with salt, pepper, and cook for 10 minutes, then turn

off.

8. When the water has come to a boil, add the gnocchi.

9. Cook them until they have all come to the surface, then drain and put them in the pan with the mushrooms.

10. Stir and then add the raw tomato cubes.

11. Stir again, put on plates and serve.

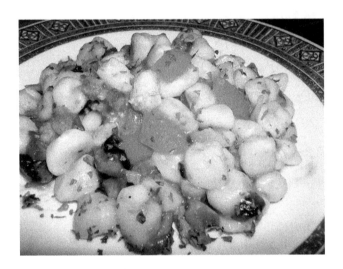

Potato gnocchi with mushrooms and saffron

PREPARATION TIME: 20 minutes

COOKING TIME: 30 minutes
CALORIES: 304

INGREDIENTS FOR 4 SERVINGS
- 600 grams of homemade potato gnocchi
-
- 2 sachets of saffron
- 250 grams of mushrooms
- 1 shallot
- 1 clove of garlic
- 125 ml of soymilk cream
- A sprig of chopped parsley
- Olive oil to taste
- Salt and Pepper to taste

DIRECTIONS
1. Bring a saucepan of water and salt to a boil.
2. Meanwhile, prepare the mushrooms. Remove the earthy part, wash them under running water and dry them. Now cut them into slices.
3. Peel and wash the garlic and shallots and then chop them.
4. Put a tablespoon of olive oil in a pan and then put the garlic and shallot to brown.
5. When they are golden brown, add the mushrooms. Stir and

season with salt, pepper, and cook for 5 minutes.

6. Put the saffron sachet in the cream and mix.

7. Now add the cream to the mushrooms and cook for another 4 minutes, stirring occasionally.

8. When the water comes to a boil, cook the gnocchi. When the gnocchi have all risen to the surface, drain and put them in the pan with the mushrooms.

9. Stir to flavour well, sauté them for a minute and then turn off.

10. Put the gnocchi on the plate, sprinkle with the chopped parsley and serve.

Potato gnocchi with peppers and cherry tomatoes

PREPARATION TIME: 20 minutes
COOKING TIME: 30 minutes

CALORIES: 267

INGREDIENTS FOR 4 SERVINGS

- 600 grams of homemade potato gnocchi

- 2 red peppers

- 2 yellow peppers

- 10 cherry tomatoes

- Olive oil to taste

- Salt and Pepper to taste

DIRECTIONS

1. Put water and salt in a saucepan and bring to a boil.

2. Meanwhile, prepare the peppers. Remove the cap, cut them in half and remove the seeds and white filaments. Wash them and then cut them into slices.

3. Wash the cherry tomatoes and cut them into four parts.

4. Heat a tablespoon of oil in a pan and as soon as it is hot, add the peppers.

5. Stir and cook for 10 minutes, then add the cherry tomatoes.

6. Season with salt and pepper, stir and cook for another five minutes.

7. When the water has come to a boil, cook the gnocchi.

8. As soon as all the gnocchi come to the surface, turn off and drain them,
9. Transfer them to the pan with the peppers, stir to flavour well and then put them on serving plates.
10. You can serve.

Wholemeal pasta salad with tofu, black olives

and cherry tomatoes

PREPARATION TIME: 20 minutes
COOKING TIME: 35 minutes

CALORIES: 294

INGREDIENTS FOR 4 SERVINGS

- 240 grams of wholemeal penne
- 2 tomatoes
- 100 grams of tofu
- 12 black olives
- A sprig of chopped parsley
- 4 chopped basil leaves
- Salt and pepper to taste
- A spoonful of balsamic vinegar
- Olive oil to taste

DIRECTIONS

1. Start with preparing the pasta.
2. Bring a pot of water and salt to a boil and then cook the pasta for 12 minutes,
3. Drain it, put it in a bowl and let it cool.
4. Meanwhile, rinse the tofu and pat it dry with absorbent paper.
5. Cut it into cubes and sauté it in a pan with hot olive oil for 3 minutes.

6. Wash the tomatoes and then cut them into cubes.
7. Put the tofu, tomatoes and olives in the bowl with the pasta and mix well.
8. Add the basil leaves, parsley, and mix again.
9. In a small bowl put the balsamic vinegar, two tablespoons of olive oil, salt and pepper.
10. Stir with a fork, until you have a homogeneous emulsion.
11. Season the pasta with the emulsion and mix to flavour all the ingredients well.
12. You can serve.

Wholemeal penne with pumpkin and onion

PREPARATION TIME: 10 minutes
COOKING TIME: 35 minutes

CALORIES: 315

INGREDIENTS FOR 4 SERVINGS

- 320 grams of wholemeal penne
- 200 grams of pumpkin pulp
- 1 white onion
- A sprig of rosemary
- Olive oil to taste
- Salt and pepper to taste

DIRECTIONS

1. Start by putting plenty of water and half a tablespoon of salt in a saucepan.
2. Bring to a boil.
3. Meanwhile, peel and wash the onion and then chop it.
4. Wash the pumpkin pulp and then cut it into cubes.
5. Wash and dry the rosemary sprig.
6. Put a tablespoon of olive oil in a pan and, once hot, put the onion to cook for 5 minutes.
7. Now add the rosemary and pumpkin.
8. Stir, season with salt, pepper, and cook for 20 minutes.
9. When the water has come to a boil, put the pasta to cook.
10. Cook for 12 minutes, then drain and transfer it to the pan with the

pumpkin.

11. Sauté the pasta for a minute, then turn off.

12. Remove the sprig of rosemary, put the pasta on the plates and
    serve.

Soy noodles with vegetables

PREPARATION TIME: 10 minutes
COOKING TIME: 15 minutes

CALORIES: 405

INGREDIENTS FOR 4 SERVINGS
- 300 grams of soy noodles
- 2 zucchinis
- 2 carrots
- 1 red pepper
- 2 shallots
- 30 grams of bean sprouts
- 40 grams of cashews
- 2 teaspoons of grated ginger
- Soy sauce to taste
- Olive oil to taste
- Salt and pepper to taste

DIRECTIONS
1. Wash the zucchinis and cut them into slices.
2. Peel and wash the carrots and shallots and then cut them into slices.
3. Remove the cap from the pepper, wash it, remove seeds and white filaments and then cut it into slices.
4. Wash and then drain the bean sprouts.

5. Put a tablespoon of oil in the wok, once hot, sauté the shallots, carrots and pepper.
6. Cook for a couple of minutes and then add the zucchinis and bean sprouts.
7. Mix well, sauté for another 2 minutes and then add the cashews.
8. Now add the ginger and two tablespoons of soy sauce.
9. The vegetables must be crunchy, then continue cooking for another 3 minutes, season with salt and pepper and turn off.
10. Now cook the spaghetti. Bring the water to a boil with salt and turn off when it boils. Pour in the soy noodles, cover with a lid and cook like this for 10 minutes.
11. Drain the soy noodles and put them in the wok with the vegetables.
12. Stir so that all the ingredients are well flavoured.
13. Now put the spaghetti on the plates and serve.

Wholemeal spaghetti with saffron and pumpkin

PREPARATION TIME: 25 minutes
COOKING TIME: 25 minutes

CALORIES: 316

INGREDIENTS FOR 4 SERVINGS

- 320 grams of wholemeal spaghetti
- 2 sprigs of rosemary
- 2 sachets of saffron
- 1 tablespoon of capers
- Olive oil to taste
- Salt and Pepper to taste

DIRECTIONS

1. Start with preparing the pasta. Bring the water and salt to a boil and cook the spaghetti for 10 minutes.
2. Meanwhile, wash and dry the rosemary and then take only the needles and throw away the branch.
3. Heat two tablespoons of oil in a pan and as soon as it is hot, add the rosemary needles to sauté.
4. Sauté them for 2 minutes and then add the capers.
5. Mix and season with salt and pepper.
6. Now drain the pasta and put a ladle of the cooking juices in a glass.
7. Put the saffron to dissolve in the glass and the pasta in the pan

with the rosemary.

8. Mix the pasta and then add the saffron.

9. Mix well until the saffron is well incorporated and turn off.

10. Put the pasta on the plates and serve.

Wholemeal tagliatelle with pumpkin and mushrooms

PREPARATION TIME: 25 minutes
COOKING TIME: 45 minutes

CALORIES: 515

INGREDIENTS FOR 4 SERVINGS

- 400 grams of wholemeal tagliatelle
- 400 grams of pumpkin
- 100 grams of mushrooms
- 1 shallot
- 250 ml of soymilk cream
- A sprig of chopped parsley
- Salt and Pepper to taste
- Olive oil to taste

DIRECTIONS

1. Put water and salt in a saucepan and bring to a boil.
2. Meanwhile, prepare the pumpkin. Peel it, remove the seeds, then wash, and cut the pulp into cubes.
3. Peel and wash the shallot and then chop finely.
4. Wash and dry the mushrooms and then cut them into slices.
5. Put a tablespoon of olive oil in a pan and as soon as it is hot, add the shallot.
6. When the shallot is wilted, add the pumpkin.
7. Stir, season with salt and pepper and then add half a glass of water.

8. Cover with a lid and cook the pumpkin for 10 minutes.

9. After 10 minutes, with the help of a fork, mash the pumpkin and then add the mushrooms.

10. Cook for another 5 minutes.

11. Meanwhile, cook the pasta for 10 minutes.

12. After 10 minutes, drain and put it in the pan with the pumpkin.

13. Add the cream, mix and cook for a couple of minutes.

14. Turn off, put the pasta on the plates and serve.